SANDRA MAHUT

Craving

EATING WELL THROUGHOUT YOUR PREGNANCY

"FABULOUS RECIPES FOR PREGNANCY, BREASTFEEDING AND BEYOND."

Photography by Émilie Guelpa

MURDOCH BOOKS

SYDNEY · LONDON

PREFACE

Yes, you can develop a craving for strawberries! I noticed it all through my pregnancy and with my pregnant friends as well. When asked what they craved during pregnancy, everyone will have their own answer. Chips, drinking yoghurt, stew, gherkins… chalk! I've heard everything!

Being pregnant means being more sensitive to your body's needs than usual and, when it comes to food, the interest in food can become obsessive! Personally, I thought about nothing but eating for all nine months of my pregnancy. I wanted everything, and different types of foods every day. I started putting together mixed plates of all kinds of things because the cravings were very real.

At the same time, you will likely hear all through your pregnancy that you mustn't eat this, or you should stay away from that. There are a few no-nos and recommendations, not to mention principles of precaution. It can be a bit of an obstacle course. Why is it important to eat well? Because your body is turning into a super baby-making machine, and food is key to the healthy development of the foetus and the resulting baby. But there is still plenty you can eat and enjoy.

I wanted to write this book to help mums-to-be satisfy their cravings, worry-free, at a time when food is so important. Don't spend your pregnancy eating tasteless cheeses and overcooked mince. With the right information, you can go to your friend's place for dinner and not be stuck eating potatoes. I've worked out some compromises, easy swaps and helpful tips to help you recreate flavours that are off-limits for the moment, but that you might be craving. Being pregnant doesn't mean being on a diet, so I've done my best to answer the many food-related questions that crop up with pregnancy. There are lots of simple recipes that are full of good things for you and your future baby, during each trimester. There are also lots of tips for staying guilt-free when dipping your spoon into a chocolate lava cake or biting into a big hamburger.

Your body is your greatest ally. It deserves to be pampered.

Sandra

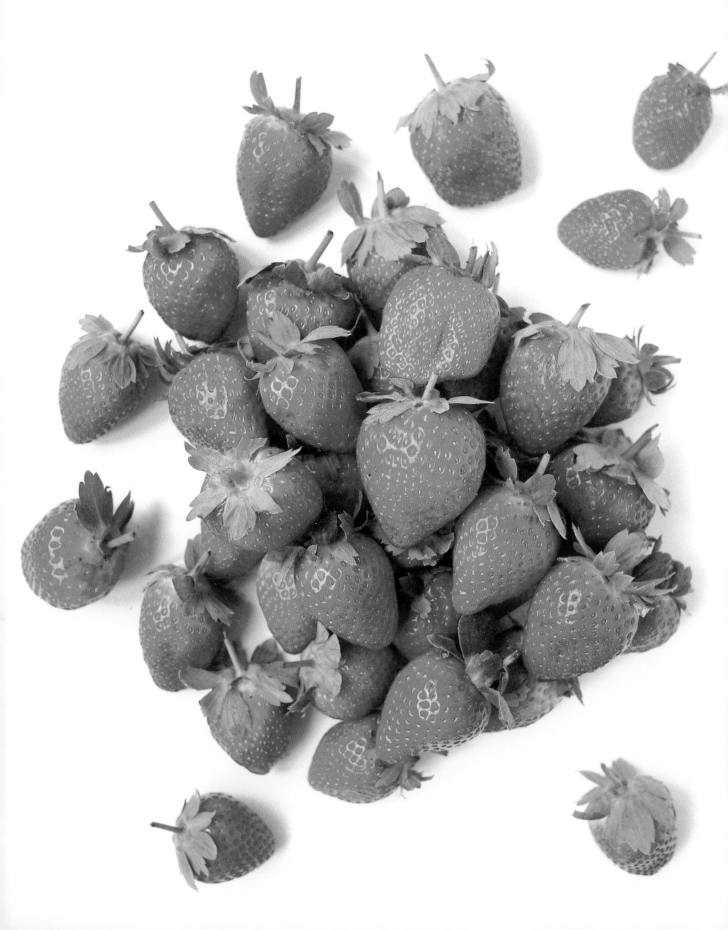

Contents

Introduction

THE PREGNANT WOMAN'S KITCHEN

Throughout your pregnancy, you'll find that your body is an amazing and very well-oiled machine. If you eat a varied and balanced diet, your baby will have all it needs to be healthy. Here are some helpful tips for developing good eating habits.

- Eat enough, but not too much! The old adage 'eating for two' is true in that you *do* need to take your own needs into account, as well as those of your unborn baby. But this doesn't mean you need to eat as much food as two fully-grown adults.

- Eat a healthy and balanced diet. This is the time to take up or return to good eating habits and eat good-quality foods.

- Eat within the guidelines provided by the medical professionals caring for you. Food guidelines and restrictions during pregnancy can vary from state to state and country to country, so educate yourself as early in your pregnancy as possible, and do your best to follow the guidelines. Taking care of yourself and your baby also means avoiding any risk of infection or intoxication. You will have to come to terms with a few temporary bans but the benefits far outweigh any frustration you may feel.

- Eat what you crave, as long as it is safe to do so. Learn how to listen to your instincts and how to indulge yourself so you sail through the next nine months feeling happy and satisfied.

Areas of precaution and foods to avoid

Certain illnesses can be dangerous to pregnant women. Because of that, some foods are off-limits for the time being.

Golden rules

In addition to the lists that follow, here are a few simple, but very important guidelines to follow when pregnant.
- No alcohol
- No smoking
- Check all medication with your obstetrician, midwife or GP to ensure it is safe to take during pregnancy.
- Eat clean, fresh and well-cooked food. If in doubt, don't eat it. You will only worry if you do.
- Always wash your hands before preparing and eating food.
- Wash fruit and vegetables well before eating.
- Ensure chopping boards (especially wooden ones) and all cooking utensils are clean when preparing food.
- Avoid cold sliced meats, soft-serve ice creams, pâtés, raw seafood, prepared salads and cheeses such as brie, camembert, feta and ricotta.
- Avoid foods that have been heated in a bain marie.
- Always wear gloves when gardening and changing cat litter trays. Wash hands properly after removing gloves.

Illnesses

During pregnancy, the immune system is a little weaker than usual and you are more vulnerable to seasonal infections, such as colds. Apart from these standard ailments, some illnesses that are normally mild can be serious for the foetus. The aim is to avoid these by cutting out consumption of risky foods, or consuming them in moderation.

Listeriosis

Listeriosis is an infection caused by the *Listeria* bacterium. In a healthy individual, it often passes unnoticed but it can be serious for young children, pregnant women and those with a compromised immune system. The illness can pass through the placental barrier and reach the foetus, so it is important to be very vigilant during pregnancy.

The bacterium is found in the environment (e.g. water, soil, plants), and in animals that ingest it. It is resistant to cold but not heat, which is why raw foods especially need to be avoided. It can be killed by cooking food to boiling point. If you reheat food, ensure it is piping hot all the way through.

PRECAUTIONS AND FOODS TO AVOID:
- raw (unpasteurised) milk, raw milk cheeses and other raw milk products
- commercial pre-packaged grated cheeses
- raw or undercooked fish, shellfish, crustaceans and meats
- marinated or smoked fish, shellfish, crustaceans and meats (unless they are cooked)
- surimi (imitation crab), fish eggs
- raw or semi-cooked cured meats
- raw or undercooked eggs and dishes that contain them.

FURTHER INFORMATION
- Some cheeses (e.g. mozzarella, camembert) are available as both pasteurised and unpasteurised versions. Check the packaging before depriving yourself.
- Whatever the type of cheese, remove the rind.
- Mass-produced egg-based dishes don't carry any risk because they use industrial "egg product" and not fresh eggs.

Toxoplasmosis

Toxoplasmosis is a common infection caused by the parasite *Toxoplasma gondii*. It's possible that you've already been exposed to the infection — most people infected don't experience any symptoms, and are immune to it after that. The risk of contamination increases considerably during pregnancy. Lesions on the foetus caused by the disease can vary in seriousness depending on its stage of development.

The infectious parasite for toxoplasmosis is present in the environment. If you are not immune to the disease, you need to limit contact with soil and wear gloves for gardening or changing cat litter.

A blood test is usually done at the beginning of pregnancy to test if you have had contact with toxoplasmosis, and are therefore immune. If you are not immune, you will continue to be monitored for nine months. Confirm with your doctor that this test has been carried out, if you are unsure.

PRECAUTIONS AND FOODS TO AVOID:

- Wash fruits, vegetables, mushrooms and herbs well to make sure there are no traces of soil left. When in doubt, eat them cooked.
- Avoid raw, undercooked, smoked or marinated meat (unless fully cooked) and cook your meat medium or well-done.

Salmonellosis

Salmonellosis is an infection caused by the *Salmonella* bacterium. It is one of the main causes of food poisoning. The illness affects the digestive system and won't have a direct effect on the foetus, but can affect you badly and make you weaker. The bacteria is found in raw foods or foods that have not been handled safely.

PRECAUTIONS AND FOODS TO AVOID:

- raw or undercooked eggs
- raw, undercooked, smoked or marinated meat
- raw milk cheeses
- wash all foods (including fruits and vegetables) and utensils that have been in contact with raw meat.

COMMENT

All methods of preparation that involve semi-cooking foods at a low temperature (foie gras, pâtés), drying, smoking, marinating, etc. don't destroy diseases and parasites. This is why it is recommended to always eat fresh foods that are well-cooked, or well-washed if raw. When in doubt about a food or how it has been prepared, don't eat it.

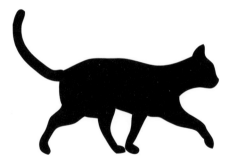

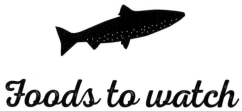

Foods to watch

For nine months, there are some foods and drinks you will have to steer clear of, and some you should only eat in moderation.

Alcohol: a no-no during pregnancy

The current recommendation is simple: don't consume any alcohol once you suspect you are pregnant. Alcohol passes through the placenta and directly affects the foetus. It can also lead to deficiencies in the pregnant woman and disturb the baby's development. Premature or smaller babies are seen at birth in women who have consumed alcohol, even in moderate quantities. No more cosmopolitans or mojitos, wine or beer while waiting for the birth. You will have lots of occasions to raise your glass in a few months!

NOTE

Alcohol can remain in a dish or dessert after it has been cooked. Depending on the cooking method, the residual amount of alcohol can vary a great deal. You can expect about 60 per cent of the initial amount of alcohol to remain in the case of a brief cooking method, such as flambéing or soaking, as in a crêpe or rum baba, and up to 10 per cent of the initial level of alcohol for a slow-cooked dish such as a beef bourguignon.

Coffee and tea

Good news, you don't have to say goodbye to your morning tea or coffee! However, it is recommended that you monitor how much caffeine you consume in a day, especially since tolerance to caffeine can vary a lot from one individual to another.

On average, the recommendation is to limit your daily consumption to 200 mg per day for a pregnant woman, which is about two coffees or two teas. Note that dark and milk chocolate also contain caffeine, but in small quantities.

Be careful with soft drinks, which, aside from containing lots of sugar, can also often contain caffeine. Read the label carefully and consume in moderation.

WHAT ARE THE RISKS WITH CAFFEINE?

- The whole attraction of caffeine, as you know, is that it stimulates the nervous system! Pregnancy can make you more sensitive to caffeine, so there's an increased risk of heart palpitations or sleeping problems for pregnant women.
- Coffee stimulates the secretion of acid in the stomach, so it can aggravate some pregnancy-related problems, like heartburn.
- Consuming too much caffeine can also be harmful to the growth of the foetus.

Fish

Because of their high levels of mercury, there are some fish you should avoid eating or only eat in moderation during pregnancy. While the tolerance threshold is rarely reached even in those who eat fish very regularly, it is better to vary the kinds of fish you eat, giving preference to oily fish. For the fish that should be consumed in moderation, allow yourself 150 g (5½ oz) per week.

- The most contaminated fish to avoid: shark (flake), swordfish, marlin.
- Contaminated fish to eat in moderation: orange roughy (deep sea perch), catfish, bonito, eel, mullet, skate, tuna.

WHAT ARE THE RISKS?

In high doses, mercury has effects on the human nervous system, especially during its development *in utero*.

Liver and offal

Liver is very high in vitamin A, and we know that very high doses of vitamin A can be harmful to the foetus. It is impossible however to reach this dosage through food, especially since liver is generally quite a small part of most people's diets. As a precaution, though, it is recommended to avoid liver and derived products.

Regarding offal meats in general, even though they are a good source of iron and folic acid, limit your intake as they are very high in vitamin A.

Soy

Soy contains phytoestrogens, which are similar to estradiol, the female sex hormone. There are currently no studies that prove consuming soy leads to hormonal disturbances. However, as a precaution, it is recommended you don't eat more than one soy-based product per day. So if you like soy milk or tofu burgers, you can keep eating them by alternating them with other kinds of protein.

Soy is a good source of plant protein if you follow a vegetarian diet. If you are in the habit of consuming more soy than the recommended dose, discuss it with your doctor, who will guide you as to what diet would suit you best.

Bad calories

Being pregnant is a good time to pick up or go back to good eating habits, with the special added motivation of doing it both for yourself and your baby.

Generally, calories are called "bad" (or "empty") when they don't provide any essential nutrients. This is especially the case with mass-produced foods that are high in simple carbohydrates, salt and saturated fats (such as mass-produced sweets, biscuits and ready-made meals). They raise blood sugar and increase the risk of cholesterol, two things to watch out for during pregnancy (see page 15). On top of that, they only give you a very brief sensation of fullness and are of course less attractive in nutritional terms. Making home-cooked meals and eating fresh foods as much as possible also guarantees that you know what you are eating and are avoiding additives and preservatives that your baby doesn't need.

That said, there is no denying the pleasure of popping a piece of confectionery in your mouth and the practical benefits of ready-made dishes for an express meal. It's not a question of depriving yourself completely of these products, just of having them occasionally.

WHAT ARE THE RISKS WITH BAD CALORIES?
- Can lead to complications for the mother (e.g. diabetes, high blood pressure, excess weight).
- Affects the development of the foetus and the growth of the future child.
- Development of gestational diabetes (see page 19).
- Increased cholesterol risks.

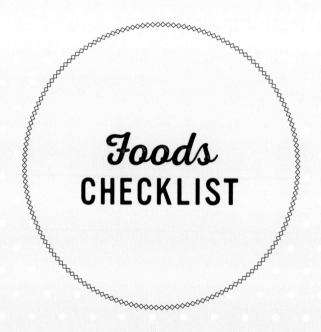

Foods
CHECKLIST

Off-limits

DAIRY PRODUCTS
- Raw (unpasteurised) milk cheeses (e.g. French brie, camembert, roquefort, Swiss gruyère) — see p. 8
- Commercial grated cheese (e.g. tasty, mozzarella) — see p. 8

FISH & FISH EGGS
- Smoked fish (smoked salmon, etc.) — see p. 8
- Raw fish (sushi, carpaccio, ceviche) — see p. 8
- Surimi (imitation crab) — see p. 8
- Taramasalata, lumpfish roe, caviar — see p. 8
- Stingray, shark (flake), swordfish — see p. 10

SHELLFISH & CRUSTACEANS
- Raw shellfish (oysters, scallop crudo, etc.) — see p. 8
- Raw crustaceans (prawn tartare, etc.) — see p. 8

MEAT
- Smoked and dried meats and products (raw ham, salami, etc.) — see p. 8–9
- Meats and dishes slow-cooked at low temperatures (rillettes, pâtés, foie gras, etc.) — see p. 8–9
- Raw or marinated meats and dishes (carpaccio, steak tartare, rare duck breast, etc.) — see p. 8–9
- Liver (calf's liver etc.) — see p. 11

EGGS
- Raw eggs and dishes containing raw eggs (home-made mayonnaise, home-made ice cream, home-made chocolate mousse, etc.) — see p. 8
- Semi-cooked eggs and dishes that contain them (e.g soft-boiled eggs, chocolate lava cakes) — see p. 8

DRINKS
- Alcohol (in drinks, but also in dishes such as flambéed crêpes, baked Alaska, rum baba) — see p. 10
- Energy drinks — see p. 18

Allowed

DAIRY PRODUCTS
- Pasteurised milk cheeses (check on the packaging): feta, mozzarella, gouda, havarti, cream cheeses — see p. 16
- Medium-hard to hard cheeses: parmesan, pecorino, comté (French gruyère), emmental — see p. 16
- Cooked (not just melted) cheeses — see p. 16

FISH
- Tinned tuna, salmon, ocean trout, trout, flounder, herring, mackerel, hake (cooked) — see p. 15

MEAT
- Cooked meats (cooked ham, sausages, meat in general)

EGGS
- Egg products (e.g. mass-produced mayonnaise, mass-produced ice cream, mass-produced chocolate mousse) — see p. 8
- Cooked eggs and dishes that contain them (hard-boiled eggs, quiche, cakes, etc.)

FRUITS & VEGETABLES
- Cooked vegetables — see p. 9
- Cooked fruits — see p. 9

Eat in moderation

FISH
- Orange roughy (deep sea perch), catfish, bonito, eel, mullet, skate, tuna (cooked) — see p. 10
- Cooked shellfish (mussels, oysters, etc.) — see p. 8
- Cooked crustaceans (prawns, crab, etc.) — see p. 8
- Cooked smoked fish

MEAT
- Offal (except liver) — see p. 11

FRUITS & VEGETABLES
- Raw vegetables — see p. 9, 23
- Herbs — see p. 9
- Raw fruit — see p. 9, 23
- Soy — see p. 11

DRINKS
- Sparkling water — see p. 21
- Tea, coffee — see p. 10
- Herbal teas — see p. 21
- Sodas and soft drinks — see p. 21

Recommended intakes

Required nutritional intakes vary according to each woman's body type and physical activity. In most cases, a balanced and varied diet will meet the nutritional needs of you and your foetus.

Quantity and quality

Pay attention to quantities and calorie intake: a woman who engages in moderate physical activity needs about 8370 kj/day (2000 cal/day). During pregnancy, these calorie requirements increase from the 2nd trimester.

- 1st trimester: 8370 kj/day (2000 cal/day).
- 2nd trimester: 9000–9200 kj/day (2150–2200 cal/day), or the equivalent of 1 apple and 1 slice of wholemeal (whole-wheat) bread extra.
- 3rd trimester: 10460 kj/day (2500 cal/day), or the equivalent of 1 muesli bar, 1 fruit salad and 1 slice of wholemeal bread extra.

Don't be overly strict when it comes your diet, which will only lead to frustration, or over indulgence. The right balance is specific to each individual. Talk about it with your doctor if necessary.

Regarding quality and nutritional intake: most of your needs only increase slightly during pregnancy. On the other hand, it is very important to have some of everything!

WHOLE FOODS / REFINED FOODS

Refined foods are often white, standardised and mass-produced. While the refinement process makes them very useful when food supplies are low (because they have a long shelf life), they lose most of their nutrients. Without demonising them, they are not considered as attractive as semi-refined or unrefined foods, which are less processed and higher in nutrients. Pregnancy can be a good time to make a few changes in your daily food choices.

Some examples:
– traditional white bread vs wholemeal (whole-wheat) or sourdough bread;
– white flour vs wholemeal (whole-wheat) flour
– pasta vs semi-wholemeal or wholemeal (whole-wheat) pasta;
– white rice vs brown rice

Everyday protein

Proteins are involved in most cellular functions; they are necessary for building and maintaining your body. Protein requirements increase gradually during pregnancy, up to 15–20% more in relation to the usual requirements during the last month. It is important therefore to eat proteins every day.

There are two types of proteins: animal proteins (found in eggs, meat, fish) and plant proteins (found in grains, legumes, nuts).

In a diet without any animal proteins, you need to eat a wide variety of plant proteins every day. If you are a vegetarian, ask your doctor for advice.

FOODS HIGH IN PROTEIN:

Animal proteins
Meat:
- beef
- turkey
- chicken
Fish:
- cod (Murray cod, blue-eye trevalla)
- red mullet
- salmon

Plant proteins
- lentils
- dried legumes
- sunflower and pepitas (pumpkin seeds)
- almonds
- tofu (see page 11 about soy products).

Remember to take quantities into account: you don't eat as much meat as sunflower seeds.

Lipids, an essential ingredient

Yes, lipids are fats, but they are essential for your body's system. They provide energy and fatty acids that are essential for cell development, and also carry several vitamins (A, D, E and K). Different types of fatty acid have different effects on our health and are more or less necessary for our body's balance.

The fatty acids to prioritise are the essential fatty acids that the body can't manufacture itself, namely the omega-3 and omega-6 fatty acids, as well as the monounsaturated fatty acids, the omega-9s.

Some foods that are especially high in essential and monounsaturated fatty acids:

For the omega-3s:
• oily fish (such as salmon, sardines, mackerel, trout)
• seeds (such as linseed), nuts.

For the omega-6s:
• vegetable oils (such as canola, sunflower, walnut, hazelnut, grapeseed, argan, sesame).

For the omega-9s:
• avocado
• olive oil.

THE DIFFERENT SUGARS

If you are watching your blood sugar levels or simply want to vary your sources of sugar, it is worth trying different sweetening agents. They can be more beneficial from a nutritional point of view and add flavour to your cooking.

– *Low glycaemic index:* agave syrup, coconut sugar.
– *Medium glycaemic index:* cane sugar (natural brown or raw [demerara] sugar), whole cane sugar (rapadura), honey, maple syrup.
– *High glycaemic index:* white refined sugar, commercial soft brown sugar.

Carbohydrates, energy to the max

Carbohydrates are our main source of energy. During pregnancy, changes in your metabolism can lead to problems with hypoglycaemia (low blood sugar). It is therefore important not to neglect carbohydrates, which provide the necessary sustained energy to the foetus (watch out all the same for gestational diabetes, see page 19).

Foods can be compared according to their glycaemic index, which is to say the way they affect blood sugar levels: when we eat a food with a high glycaemic index, the blood sugar level rises rapidly and we release a lot of insulin. If we eat a food with a low glycaemic index, the blood sugar level rises slowly and less insulin is released.

Insulin is the "storing" hormone. A slow release will give the body time to burn the carbohydrates, while a quick release will often mean the carbohydrates are stored.

Some foods with a low glycaemic index:
• whole grains (such as barley, burghul [bulgur], rice, quinoa)
• legumes (chickpeas, lentils, dried beans, broad beans)
• green vegetables, berries, nuts in general.

Some foods with a high glycaemic index:
• white breads; white rice
• confectionery, sugars in general.

Some false friends:
• puffed rice cakes
• dates.

THE CASE OF FIBRE

Fibre is part of the carbohydrate family. Derived from plants, it is essential for the digestive system to function properly. It is especially useful during pregnancy, when the digestive system often slows down.

Some especially high-fibre foods:
• legumes (such as dried beans, lentils, kidney beans, peas, chickpeas)
• the cabbage family
• artichokes, leeks, fennel
• berries (e.g. raspberries, blackcurrants, blackberries)
• wholemeal (whole-wheat) bread, whole grains
• nuts

Recommended intakes

Vitamins and minerals.

Essential minerals

CALCIUM, FOR YOU AND YOUR BABY

Calcium preserves your bone mass. During pregnancy, it is essential for making the foetus' bones and teeth. Plus, calcium reduces the risk of high blood pressure for the future mother, as well as the risk of the baby blues! In short, it's a good time to indulge in some (pasteurised) cheese therapy.

Normally our daily needs are 700 mg calcium per day. It is very important to reach this target every day by eating 2 or 3 serves of dairy products, combining them with other plant and animal foods that are high in calcium.

1 x 150 ml (5 fl oz) yoghurt = 225 mg calcium
1 x 30 g (1 oz) serve of cheese = 220 mg calcium
1 x 125 ml (4 fl oz/½ cup) cow's milk = 180 mg calcium

Calcium is, of course, found in dairy products, but if these make you feel nauseous early in the pregnancy, there are several plant foods that also contain calcium.

Some especially high-calcium foods:
• milk and dairy products (yoghurt, cheese)
• tinned fish
• almonds
• dried figs
• fresh parsley, thyme
• the cabbage family (try kale, broccoli, brussels sprouts)
• pepitas (pumpkin seeds)
• some mineral waters.
Remember to take quantities into account: you don't eat as many pumpkin seeds as yoghurt.

IRON, TO AVOID DEFICIENCIES

Iron plays an important role in several vital functions. During pregnancy, there is a significant rise in your total blood volume, which logically leads to increased iron needs. Daily iron consumption contributes to the formation of a healthy placenta, a good level of red blood cells and will also help fight against fatigue due to anaemia.

Since nature is smart, it improves the body's absorption of iron during pregnancy. Nevertheless, a blood test during the first trimester will determine whether you need a supplement.

You will be advised in any case to take an iron supplement during the last trimester, especially to avoid any deficiencies at the time of delivery. Iron is found in red meat, but also white meat, fish and eggs. Those who don't eat much meat need to look to dried legumes and green vegetables.

Comment
Time your tea! It significantly reduces iron absorption. So avoid taking your iron supplement while drinking tea. Instead, try taking it with a fresh fruit juice, since vitamin C improves iron absorption.

Some especially high-iron foods:
• meat (such as beef, chicken, pork, lamb, black pudding)
• eggs
• broccoli, kale, watercress
• legumes (lentils, chickpeas, etc.)
• wholemeal (whole-wheat) bread and whole grains
• dried fruit and nuts
• chocolate.
Remember to take into account the amounts you consume: you don't eat as much chocolate as meat (at least in theory).

OTHER MINERALS: SALT, IODINE, ETC.

Your needs in salt, iodine and other minerals like magnesium or phosphorous are usually easily covered by a varied diet. If you are anaemic or have a specific deficiency or condition, your doctor may prescribe a supplement for you.

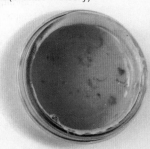

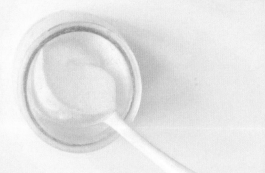

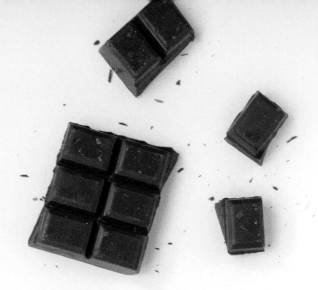

Pregnancy-specific vitamins

FOLIC ACID (OR FOLATES, VITAMIN B9), FOR THE NERVOUS SYSTEM

Folic acid (or Vitamin B9) is vital during the early months of pregnancy because it enables the growth and development of tissue. Your needs increase by about a third. A deficiency can seriously affect the baby's nervous system and brain development. For this reason, a folic acid supplement is recommended as soon as you start trying for a baby, then at the beginning of the pregnancy. VItamin B9 is found in the leaves of certain vegetables and nuts.

Some foods that are especially high in folic acid:
- salad greens (such as watercress, mâche, witlof [chicory], dandelion, rocket [arugula])
- green vegetables (such as green beans, peas, broccoli, spinach)
- legumes (lentils, beans, chickpeas)
- some cheeses (such as blue cheese, if pasteurised)
- citrus fruits (grapefruit, orange)
- walnuts and chestnuts.

VITAMIN D, TO BOOST CALCIUM

Vitamin D allows the body to absorb and use calcium. Given the need for calcium during pregnancy, it is very important. Apart from some oily fish and dairy products, not much vitamin D is found in food. On the other hand, the body manufactures it itself by synthesising sunlight on the skin. It is therefore important to get outside on a regular basis, but this isn't always enough and pregnant women often have a deficiency. A supplement is often prescribed, especially when the pregnancy occurs during winter when the sunlight is weak.

Some foods that are especially high in vitamin D:
- some fish (like salmon, herring, tuna, sardines, mackerel) (see page 10 about fish choices)
- butter, egg yolk (well cooked)
- whole milk.

Other vitamins

Except in special cases, your needs for other vitamins (A, B, C, E, K) are covered by a balanced diet.

Water!

Drink (water) freely during pregnancy. It is usually recommended that adults drink about 1.5 litres (52 fl oz/6 cups) per day and this also applies during pregnancy. The foetus' need for water increases as it develops and drinking water contributes to the amniotic fluid. At the end of pregnancy, this amounts to almost 1 litre (35 fl oz/4 cups). Drinking enough water also plays a preventative role when it comes to urinary infections and constipation, which are common during pregnancy.

WHY CHOOSE ORGANIC?

Eating organic foods involves a number of broader questions: accessibility, extra cost, the environment, food provenance… which we can't discuss here.

Given some chemical substances can pass through the placental barrier and reach the foetus, we can however point out that regulations are stricter for organic foods:
– when it comes to treating fresh and processed foods;
– when it comes to added preservatives, colours and additives.

Choose organic:
– *for fruits and vegetables.* Find out whether they undergo a lot of treatments during production; this is especially important if you eat the skin.
– *for meat, eggs and dairy products,* because some intensive farming uses antibiotics and hormone treatments that can be found in these products.
– *for whole dried goods,* because grains can store pesticides in their husk.

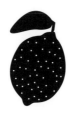

Good habits and myths

*There are some simple things to keep in mind
and a few common preconceptions to forget.*

Good habits

FRESH, GOOD QUALITY FOODS

This is obvious at any time in your life, and should be even more so when you are pregnant: pay attention to the freshness and quality of foods. Pay special attention to seafoods: you can eat them cooked without any worry if you are quite sure of their freshness. Food poisoning doesn't happen often, but if you have the smallest doubt, it's better to abstain.

HYGIENE REMINDER

- Wash your hands after contact with raw foods (meat, vegetables, etc.) and wash well any surfaces (chopping boards, kitchen benches) that have been in contact with these foods, to limit the risks of food poisoning and transmitting disease (see page 8).
- Clean your fridge regularly and adhere to expiry dates.
- Be careful to respect the cold food chain for perishables: thaw food properly by placing it in the refrigerator the night before using; never refreeze a frozen product.

NATURAL CLEANING PRODUCTS

Try using natural products for cleaning. In addition to being better for the environment, you will avoid breathing in toxic substances. To effectively clean your refrigerator, fill a spray bottle with 50% water and 50% white vinegar, and add a little lemon juice to deodorise. White vinegar is inexpensive, disinfects and prevents mould.

Myths

SWEETENERS

Pregnant women don't need to consume "lite" or diet foods, because they are trying to get as much energy as possible from their diet. There is no benefit to eating diet foods during pregnancy in the context of a balanced diet.

During pregnancy, the dangers of consuming aspartame, other artificial sweeteners or derived products that contain them (soft and energy drinks or desserts) are not currently proven. Even so, water is still the best choice. If you are in the habit of drinking diet soft drinks, limit them to 1 or 2 per week.

On the other hand, the natural sweetener stevia can be used in place of sugar (especially if you have gestational diabetes), but still in moderate quantities.

Note

If you are watching your sugar intake because of gestational diabetes, you should prefer "alternative sugars" with a low glycaemic index (see page 10). Ask your doctor for advice.

MASS-PRODUCED "FUNCTIONAL FOODS"

Mass-produced "functional foods", which is to say processed foods with claimed medical benefits, such as special anti-cholesterol products, are of no use to pregnant women. Choose healthy, simple and varied foods and they will meet your nutritional needs.

Depending on your needs, vitamin-enriched fortified foods (enriched milk, for example), can be worthwhile during pregnancy.

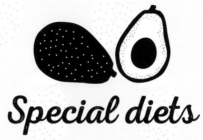

Special diets

Keep in mind that during pregnancy,
everything is about balance.

Gestational diabetes

Gestational diabetes mellitus (GDM) or pregnancy-related diabetes is a problem with the regulation of blood sugar, leading to an increase in the sugar levels in the blood. It emerges during the second or third trimester and usually disappears after pregnancy.

Certain factors can predispose you to diabetes: being an older mother, being overweight or having a family history of Type 2 diabetes can mean you are more likely to develop GDM. Ethnic background can also play a role: Middle Eastern, Vietnamese, Chinese, Indian, African and Polynesian or Melanesian women, for example, can be at greater risk.

Gestational diabetes can reveal itself in certain symptoms (e.g. strong thirst, tiredness), but it can also occur without any particular signs.

In any case, a pregnant woman with diabetes needs to be medically supervised, because diabetes can lead to major complications for the mother and child. Most pregnant women are given a fasting blood test for GDM around 24–28 weeks into their pregnancy.

If you have GDM, you will be monitored throughout your pregnancy, and you will also need to check your own blood glucose levels four times day. It is important to see a diabetic educator to adapt your diet to maintain moderate blood sugar levels. Generally speaking, it is a matter of:
• focusing on foods with a low glycaemic index (see page 15) and keeping a careful watch on sugars;
• choosing high-fibre foods (see page 15);
• eating the right types of food regularly throughout the day, as advised by your doctor or diabetic educator.

If GDM is well controlled and you are able to keep your blood glucose in check, your levels will stay in the range for a healthy pregnancy. However, if your GDM cannot be managed by diet, you may need to take medication or insulin injections.

Vegetarian, vegan, gluten-free...

If you decide or are obliged to exclude certain types of food from your diet, it is essential for you to talk about it with your doctor, who will advise you on the best way to follow your diet during pregnancy and can prescribe you dietary supplements if needed.

At the same time, even if you aren't following any particular diet, trying out alternatives, having as much variety as possible and discovering new flavours are always avenues to explore, whether you are pregnant or not. There are several vegetarian, vegan and gluten-free recipes in this book.

Weight loss diets: in the bin

Any deficiency can be harmful to you or your baby, so this is not the time to start a weight loss diet. If you have to follow a particular diet, or suffer from weight problems, it is essential to talk about it with your doctor. (See also gestational diabetes, opposite).

Medicinal and dietary supplements

A balanced and varied diet will cover your basic needs. If necessary, some dietary supplements will be prescribed for you, depending on the stage of your pregnancy, to cover very specific needs:
• Folic Acid (Vitamin B9) (see page 17): prescribed as soon as you start planning a pregnancy and during the first weeks of your pregnancy.
• Iron (see page 16): prescribed if there are concerns about deficiencies or to prevent them.
• Vitamin D (see page 17): prescribed if blood tests done at the beginning of the pregnancy and again at 28 weeks indicate low levels of Vitamin D. If a mother is low in Vitamin D, it is advised that her baby be given drops at birth (unless formula fed, as formula includes Vitamin D).
• A pregnancy-specific multi-vitamin is advised as a daily supplement for all pregnant and breastfeeding women. These can be large tablets, so crush them into jam or purchase soluble tablets, if nauseated.

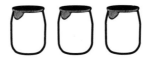

The pantry of the mum-to-be

Making balanced meals is much simpler when you have what you need on hand.
Here are a few essentials to have in your cupboards for nine months (and beyond).

GRAINS, DRIED LEGUMES, PASTA

Grains and legumes, to cook or as flakes:
- quinoa
- burghul (bulgur)
- couscous
- yellow, red and green lentils
- white, basmati and arborio rice
- rolled oats.

Pasta:
- wheat pasta, buckwheat pasta, spelt pasta, etc.
- white, semi-wholemeal, wholemeal (whole-wheat) pasta.

Dried fruits, nuts, and seeds
- almonds, hazelnuts, walnuts, pecans, macadamia nuts, pine nuts, etc.
- raisins, dried apricots, cranberries, dates, prunes, dried mango, flaked coconut
- pepitas (pumpkin seeds), linseed (flaxseed), sesame seeds, poppy seeds, sunflower seeds, etc.

NUT BUTTERS
- almond, hazelnut butter
- peanut butter.

FLOURS
- white, semi-wholemeal and wholemeal (whole-wheat) wheat flours
- non-wheat flours: buckwheat, chestnut, rye, maize, etc.

SEASONINGS, CONDIMENTS & SAUCES
- salt, gomasio (sesame seed seasoning)
- black pepper, mixed pepper, hot paprika
- standard mustard, wholegrain mustard, honey-mustard sauce
- gherkins
- soy sauce.

SUGARS
- soft brown sugar, raw (demerara) sugar
- agave syrup
- maple syrup
- thyme honey, acacia honey, etc.

TINNED FOODS
- sweet corn
- cannellini beans, kidney beans
- peeled, crushed tomatoes
- sardines, tuna, salmon.

OILS
- olive oil
- nut oils: walnut, hazelnut, etc.
- seed oils: sunflower, canola, grapeseed, etc.

MILKS
- dairy milks: cow's, goat's etc.
- plant milks (e.g. almond, oat).

IN THE FREEZER
- herbs: basil, chives, coriander (cilantro), parsley, etc.
- vegetables: spinach, broccoli, etc.
- fruits: raspberries, mixed berries, plums, rhubarb, etc.

S.O.S. SNACKS
Sweet:
- chocolate
- muesli bars
- dried fruit and nuts.

Savoury:
- multigrain crackers
- puffed rice cakes, corn cakes.

Fresh foods:
- fruits: apple, grapes
- vegetables: carrots cut into sticks, cherry tomatoes
- hard cheeses.

Drinks:
- fruit juice
- vegetable juice (carrot, tomato).

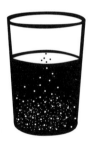

To drink

It is important to stay hydrated, especially during pregnancy. If the pregnant woman's plate is full of rich and delicious things, her glass should be as well!

WATER

This is the preferred drink on a day-to-day basis, during and between meals, it has no calories. Have a small bottle of water in your bag to drink all day.

Unless there are specific restrictions where you live (ask the local council), you can drink as much tap water as you like. You can also drink as much mineral water as you like. They each have their specific features and flavours, so try a variety. As for sparkling waters, drink them in moderation as they are often high in sodium.

FLAVOURED WATERS & CORDIALS

Without adding any sugar, you can very easily liven up water by infusing a few fruits, herbs or spices in it for 15 minutes with some ice cubes.

A few ideas:
• 1 slice of watermelon + 5 crushed basil leaves
• 5 crushed mint leaves + 1 piece of crushed ginger
• 1 slice pineapple + ½ kiwifruit.
For sweeter drinks, you can also use cordials or store-bought flavoured waters (look at the ingredients to see how much sugar they contain).

FRESH JUICES

The fresher the juice, the better it is from a nutritional point of view. Don't overdo them, though, as they still contain lots of sugar and aren't the same as eating a fresh piece of fruit.

ALCOHOL-FREE COCKTAILS (SEE PAGE 102)

Alcohol-free cocktails are special occasion drinks. Keep an eye on them, as they often contain lots of sugar.

SOFT DRINKS

Soft carbonated drinks are very high in sugar and often contain caffeine, which should be limited during pregnancy (see page 10). They should only be consumed occasionally.

TEA & COFFEE

Coffee, and to a lesser extent tea, should be limited during pregnancy (see page 10) due to their caffeine content, which is very stimulating and potentially harmful to the foetus.

MILK

High in protein, vitamin D and calcium, milk is the ally of the pregnant woman. During pregnancy, it should be pasteurised to prevent the risk of listeriosis (see page 8). Nevertheless, milk is also a high-energy food; think of it as a side to your meals, or a snack.

PLANT MILKS

Plant milks are beverages generally made from seeds, nuts or grains that have been ground and cold-filtered. Unless they are fortified, plant milks don't contain calcium and so aren't a substitute for milk in the diet of the pregnant woman. However, each plant milk has its own special nutritional properties, and its milky texture means it can be substituted for the same quantity of milk in recipes, especially in baking. They are also sweet and digestible.

HERBAL TEAS

Herbal teas offer you a hot drink in a wide variety of flavours and without added sugar. Each plant also has properties that can potentially relieve the small discomforts of pregnancy.

A few herbal teas for pregnant women:
• ginger, marjoram, lemon balm: for nausea
• red vine leaf: for swollen legs
• lavender, lemon balm, linden: for insomnia
• angelica: anti-stress.
Beware of uterotonic teas (such as raspberry or sage) that can encourage contractions, plants that can irritate the digestive system or that have a diuretic or laxative effect. Ask your doctor or pharmacist for information.

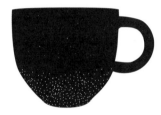

Kitchen tips

*There are lots of tricks for reducing the salt, sugar and fat in
dishes without affecting their flavour. Play with seasonings
and cooking methods for healthier and tastier dishes.*

Condiments and seasonings

SALT

- Soy sauce, a sauce made from fermented, salted and flavoured
  soy. Although it is high in salt, there are also low-salt versions,
  ideal for a marinade for example (see recipe page 162).
- Gomasio, a condiment made from ground sesame seeds
  and a small amount of salt, gives you a light seasoning while
  adding a hint of toasted sesame flavour to every dish.
- Celery salt is a condiment made from dried and ground
  celeriac and a small amount of salt, to season and give
  bite to a plate of raw vegetables or bowls of soup.
- Spices lift dishes and bring out flavours. Get
  into the habit of tasting a dish after adding
  spices, you will certainly add less salt.
- Marinades: marinating meats and fish for 30 minutes
  before cooking, in lemon juice or an oil of your choice,
  gives them flavour without adding salt. If you use
  the marinade later in the recipe, remember to heat
  it for 2 minutes to avoid any contamination.

FLAVOURS

- Smoky: use smoked salt.
- Spicy: use wasabi, Tabasco sauce.
- Herbs: try to always have a few fresh herbs (or
  else frozen or dried) in the kitchen; they give a
  finishing touch to a dish and are full of vitamins.

Fats

OILS

There are a wide variety of vegetable oils which
each have their own properties, qualities and uses.
Try varying them discover different flavours, but also
for the different nutritional benefits of each.

Some examples:

- Olive oil: high in oleic acid, which helps digestion,
  perfect for cooking or using cold.
- Canola oil: high in vitamins K and E, it is used cold or in
  cakes for a more neutral flavour (see recipe page 124).
- Sesame oil: high in antioxidants and vitamin E (see recipe
  page 110); it gives a pleasant aroma to salads and
  raw vegetables.
- Walnut oil: high in omega-3s and vitamin E, it is used cold
  for a very fruity flavour. It is ideal for salads or to dress plain
  rice or pasta.

BUTTER

Derived from milk, butter doesn't always have a good
reputation in our diet because it is very high in calories.
Nevertheless, consumed in moderation, butter is still
a good source of vitamin A and indulgence!

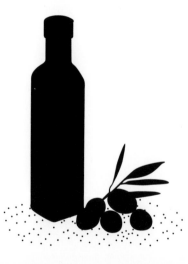

NUT BUTTERS

Nut butters are made from nuts and seeds ground into a paste. Easy to digest and with no added sugar, they are an interesting alternative to butter in lots of recipes, especially sweet ones.

Some examples

- Blanched, semi-blanched or unblanched almond pastes: made from almonds with or without their skin, they have a mild almond flavour. Use as a spread or in baking (replace softened butter with the same quantity of almond butter) (see recipes pages 62, 80, 82).
- Hazelnut butter: made from toasted hazelnuts, it has a strong hazelnut flavour. For spreading or using in baking (see recipes pages 56, 127, 133).
- Sesame paste or white or unhulled tahini: made from hulled or unhulled sesame seeds. Slightly bitter, it has a mild taste, ideal for savoury dishes (see recipes pages 41, 104, 110).

Cooking methods:

DIFFERENT WAYS OF COOKING

There are different ways of cooking food, and each method has its advantages and disadvantages. There is no ideal cooking method. To decide, you need of course to consider the health benefits and preserving the nutrients of each food. But you also have to consider day-to-day practicalities, cooking times and the addition of fat or not.

Generally speaking, quick, high-temperature cooking methods that sear foods tend to be aggressive on foods and destroy vitamins. In contrast, low-temperature cooking methods preserve nutrients.

Some guidelines

- Cooking with steam and *en papillote* (in a foil or baking paper package): a fairly quick cooking method. Preserves the vitamins, minerals and natural flavours, and requires little added fat.
- Baking, braising and stewing: slower cooking methods. The longer the cooking time and higher the temperature, the greater the loss of nutrients, flavours on the other hand are intensified;

- Microwave cooking: quick cooking time, practical for reheating. Destroys vitamins, only use occasionally;
- Grilling and barbecuing: fast cooking method. Gives unique flavours to foods and uses little added fat, but on the other hand burnt and carbonised fats form a harmful substance. To be used occasionally.

RAW

Be careful: eating raw meat and fish is not recommended during pregnancy due to the risk of food poisoning (see page 8–9).

When it comes to raw fruit and vegetables, eating these means you can take advantage of all their nutrients. When you are pregnant however, there are a few necessary precautions. Make sure you wash foods well (see page 9) and, as much as possible, pay attention to where they came from and how they were produced. Once they have been picked, fruits and vegetables lose their nutritional qualities, up to 50% of their vitamins in two or three days in the open air. Choosing seasonal and local products means you can have the freshest possible fruits and vegetables.

A few preparation ideas:

- Whole, or as raw vegetable sticks: you can munch on fresh fruits and vegetables as long as you wash them well.
- In smoothies or fresh juices: squeezing raw fruits, blending them whole or cold-extracting their juice gives you a wide variety of drinks while preserving the maximum amount of vitamins.

Getting organised

It can be challenging to eat well when you are tired and planning for the baby's arrival, and once the baby has arrived, it can be even harder! Here are a few tips for getting ready towards the end of your pregnancy.

Get ahead on prep

– Clean and dice mixed vegetables to put in a bag and freeze for making express soups, stir-fries, etc.:
• tomato soup (see page 114)
• pumpkin (squash) soup (see page 115).
– Clean, seed and dice mixed fresh fruits to put in sachets and freeze for making express compotes, sautéed fruit, express desserts:
• compote (see page 38)
• strawberry soup (see page 135).

Cooking in bulk

– Make an extra batch of cakes, let them cool completely and freeze them individually for a sweet, comforting treat:
• blueberry muffins (see page 124)
• yoghurt cupcakes (see page 125).
– Cook a family meal and let it cool completely before freezing one or several portions for an express full meal:
• make a tagine or stew (see page 149), and prepare the grain at the last moment.

Fresh, frozen, tinned

Although it is important to eat fresh foods, don't turn your back on frozen or tinned foods. They broaden your cooking options and make it even easier to vary your diet.

FRESH FOODS

This is the preferred choice for everyday eating. Apart from their nutritional qualities, they bring flavour and texture to cooking. However, to get the most out of them, remember they should be as fresh as possible. Peas for example lose up to 50% of their vitamin C one day after being picked.

FROZEN FOODS

These are a worthwhile alternative. Not all fruits and vegetables are equal when it comes to freezing, some keep their nutritional qualities very well (e.g. zucchini, artichoke hearts), other more fragile ones don't handle the cold very well (e.g. cabbages, peas). In spite of everything, this method of preservation means you can eat vegetables all year round, even out of season. Finally, we can't neglect the practical side: it is easy to make yourself a quick soup with frozen, ready-to-use vegetables.

TINNED FOODS

These often have a bad reputation because vegetables lose a lot of nutrients when preserved in this way. Also keep a close watch on added salt and even sugar, if you eat them regularly. Avoid drinking or using the liquid from tinned foods (except tomatoes) for this reason. At the same time, this method offers the longest shelf-life in the cupboard and allows products to be available at any time.

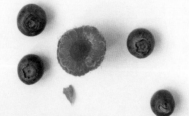

Diet and breastfeeding

Some nutritional information for mums planning to breastfeed.

Breast milk

Breast milk is a complete food, full of nutrients and easy to digest. Its composition changes as the days go by to exactly meet the baby's needs. If you choose to breastfeed, you don't need to follow a specific dietary regime, but to maintain a balanced diet and keep well hydrated.

Diet and milk quality

Your own diet doesn't affect the nutritional composition of your milk, it will always be "good". On the other hand, some things you consume can pass into your breast milk. Watch out for the following.

AVOID:
- alcohol: it passes into the breast milk
- cigarettes: nicotine passes into the breast milk
- diets: don't start a post-pregnancy diet, you will need all of your energy!

LIMIT:
- coffee and tea (see page 10) – caffeine passes into the breast milk
- "functional foods" (see page 18)
- medicines – they can pass into the breast milk. Tell your doctor that you are breastfeeding if you need to be treated for a medical condition
- peanuts (if you have an allergy, or if your baby is at risk of developing an allergy)
- fruit and fruit juices (if your baby is colicky or has diarrhoea).

CONSUME MORE:
- calcium (see page 16), take advantage of the fact that you no longer have to limit yourself to pasteurised cheeses
- vitamin D (see page 17)
- iron (see page 16)
- iodine (see page 16).

STIMULATE LACTATION:
- drink herbal teas for breastfeeding: 2–3 cups/day (some plants are said to promote lactation: fennel, star anise, fenugreek, cumin)
- eat certain foods believed to have stimulant properties: oats, barley, almonds, lentils.

MYTHS

Drinking beer during breastfeeding stimulates lactation
Some believe that malt, which is used to make beer, stimulates milk production, but the potential consequences of the baby absorbing the alcohol cancels out all the benefits. It is better to eat whole grains and sprinkle plenty of nutritional yeast on your salads.

Drinking lots of milk means you can produce more breast milk
Drinking large amounts of milk doesn't have any effect on the production of breast milk, but a lactating mother requires at least 2–3 litres of water a day. So stay hydrated!

Foods with a strong flavour like cabbage should be avoided
Strong flavours can flavour your breast milk. It is the start of your baby developing a palate for a variety of tastes. Some infants are very sensitive to it and will oblige you to limit your consumption, others will appreciate it.

Craving

First trimester
Grazing

The principle

In the first trimester, it's difficult to avoid nausea. You can't get your breakfast down in the same way. You will have to eat the same amount of food, but in a different way, to keep your energy levels up. Here are a few things to help you.

Foods to combat nausea

You may begin to crave acidic foods, like mandarins. Citrus fruits, even their scent alone, can help quell the nausea. Many women who experience nausea in the first trimester crave salty food, but this often settles down in the second and third trimesters. Eat a small amount, if necessary. And remember, what works for nausea is not a one-size-fits-all; one woman's cure may be another's undoing. The most important thing is to keep fluids up and maintain a good urine output.

Foods to combat fatigue

For the little dips in energy that happen during the day, have small bags of nuts and sesame biscuits in your handbag when you go out.

Foods to aid digestion

Herbal teas for digestion, green tea, citrus, ginger, detoxifying vegetables — all of these are good for soothing those little upsets that will pass when the second trimester arrives.

Breakfast
IDEAS
(for dipping into)

In the first trimester, you have to negotiate between the need for varied sources of nutrition and the realities of morning sickness. Here are some ideas for something different when you're in a hurry.

Craving fruit

Fruit, yes! But with the nausea that comes with the first trimester, it's generally better to choose fruits that are easier to digest and less acidic:

- well-ripened fruit, dried fruit or cooked fruit
- compote
- mashed banana
- fruity drinking yoghurts.

Craving toast

It's easy to add variety to your toast or bread and butter: this is the time to drop simple white bread and sample the wide range of delicious breads with seeds, nuts and dried fruit. Try breads made from different flours and wholemeal (whole-wheat) or semi-wholemeal breads that are have more value from a nutritional point of view, but are also much more digestible:

- fingers of multigrain bread + olive oil
- hazelnut bread + almond butter + grated square of chocolate (or almond butter and prunes puréed together)
- kamut or corn bread (gluten-free) + compote.

Craving savoury

Breakfast carbohydrates and proteins are also found in savoury foods. Think about topping your bread with pasteurised cheese or the good fats in avocado as a change from butter and jam:

- multigrain bread + ricotta (or other whey cheese) + walnut kernels
- dark rye bread + ricotta + honey + cinnamon + pepitas (pumpkin seeds)
- wholemeal (whole-wheat) bread + thin slices of avocado + agave syrup + fresh coriander (cilantro).

Craving savoury

Craving fruit

Craving toast

Anti-Nausea
BREAKFAST

*Top the ginger yoghurt with a generous tablespoon
of crunchy granola. Enjoy with the citrus salad.*

Mini citrus salad
GRAPEFRUIT + BLOOD ORANGE

MAKES 2 BOWLS
PREPARATION TIME 10 MINUTES

1 organic pink grapefruit
1 organic blood orange
½ pomegranate, seeds extracted
2 cumquats, well washed, sliced into thin rounds
4 tablespoons agave syrup
zest of ½ organic lime

Remove the rind and membrane from the grapefruit and
blood orange with a knife and discard. Slice the flesh
very thinly. Divide the grapefruit, orange, pomegranate
seeds, cumquats and lime zest between two plates.
Sprinkle with agave syrup. Chill in the refrigerator or
enjoy straight away.

Crunchy granola
HAZELNUTS + ALMONDS + SEEDS

MAKES 1 LARGE JAR
PREPARATION TIME 15 MINUTES
COOKING TIME 40 MINUTES

50 g (1¾ oz) hazelnuts + 50 g (1¾ oz) almonds
   + 50 g (1¾ oz) pecans + 50 g (1¾ oz) walnuts
200 g (7 oz) rolled oats
4 tablespoons seeds (linseed [flaxseed], sesame,
   sunflower)
2 tablespoons desiccated (shredded) coconut
½ teaspoon salt
3 tablespoons coconut oil
3–4 tablespoons honey
2 tablespoons raw (demerara) or light brown sugar

Preheat the oven to 150°C (300°F). Roughly chop the
nuts with a knife or in a food processor (1–2 pulses).

Combine all of the dry ingredients in a large mixing
bowl; season with salt. Place the coconut oil, honey
and sugar in a saucepan. Heat gently for a few
minutes, stirring.

Line a baking tray with baking paper and spread over the
mixture of dried ingredients. Pour the liquid mixture over
the top and mix well to coat the grains and nuts. Cook
in the oven for about 40 minutes; stir half way through
the cooking time. The granola should gently brown but
not burn. Let the mixture cool at room temperature.
Roughly break up the pieces then store them in a jar.

Ginger yoghurt
WITH CARDAMOM + HONEY

MAKES 6–8 SMALL TUBS
PREPARATION TIME 10 MINUTES
COOKING TIME 12 HOURS
RESTING TIME 4 HOURS

1 litre (35 fl oz/4 cups) pasteurised milk
125 g (4½ oz/1 small tub) plain yoghurt
seeds from ½ cardamom pod, husk removed
½ cm (¼ inch) fresh ginger, peeled and grated
2 teaspoons honey or agave syrup, or 3 dates (optional)

Whisk the milk with the plain yoghurt in a mixing bowl
until well combined. Crush the cardamom seeds to a
fine powder. Mix the ginger and cardamom into the
milk-yoghurt mixture. If you want to, you can sweeten
the mixture with honey, agave syrup or puréed dates.
Pour the mixture into glass yoghurt pots and place
them in a yoghurt-maker for 12 hours. Chill for at
least 4 hours in the refrigerator before serving.

TIP: The granola keeps for 2–3 weeks at room
temperature in an airtight container away from light.
The home-made yoghurts will keep for 1 week
in the refrigerator.

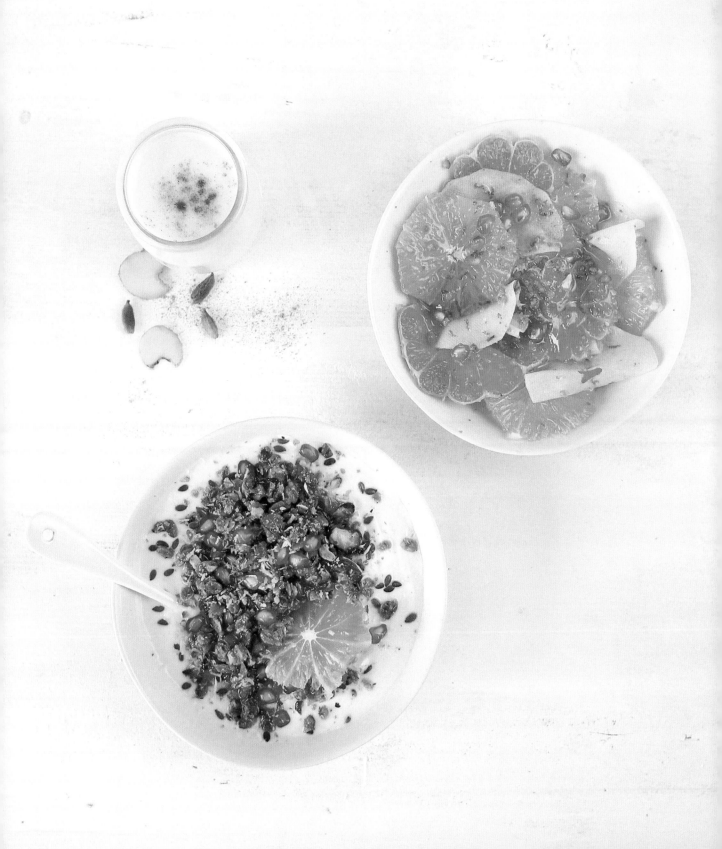

Energy
BREAKFAST

Serve still-hot French toast with a well-chilled
smoothie. A cocktail of indulgence and vitamins.

French toast
WITH BANANA + MAPLE SYRUP

MAKES 2 GENEROUS SLICES
PREPARATION TIME 10 MINUTES
COOKING TIME 5 MINUTES

1 large free-range egg
125 ml (4 fl oz/½ cup) pasteurised milk
1 vanilla bean, seeds scraped (or ½ teaspoon vanilla
    powder, or liquid vanilla extract)
2 slices stale bread or brioche
1 knob of butter, for frying
1 tablespoon muscovado sugar (or light brown,
    or raw [demerara] sugar)
1 sliced banana (or 1 handful berries, or
    another fruit of your choice, well washed)
1 tablespoon icing (confectioners') sugar
4 tablespoons maple syrup

Whisk the egg with the milk and vanilla in a large,
shallow dish. Place the bread in the mixture and turn
over to coat both sides well.

Melt a knob of butter in a frying pan and lay the soaked
bread in the pan, without the pieces touching each
other. Brown each side for a few minutes. Sprinkle with
muscovado sugar; the bread will lightly caramelise.

Place the French toast on a plate, scatter with
slices of banana, then dust with icing sugar. Lightly
drizzle with maple syrup and serve while still hot.

Blueberry smoothie
WITH KALE + ORANGE + LEMON

MAKES 2 LARGE GLASSES
PREPARATION TIME 10 MINUTES

juice of 2 organic oranges
juice of 1 organic lemon
80 g (2¾ oz) fresh (or frozen) blueberries
1 handful kale, shredded, or curly cabbage
2 tablespoons honey or agave syrup (optional)

Liquidise all of the ingredients in a blender.
Add a little water to thin out the smoothie, if necessary.

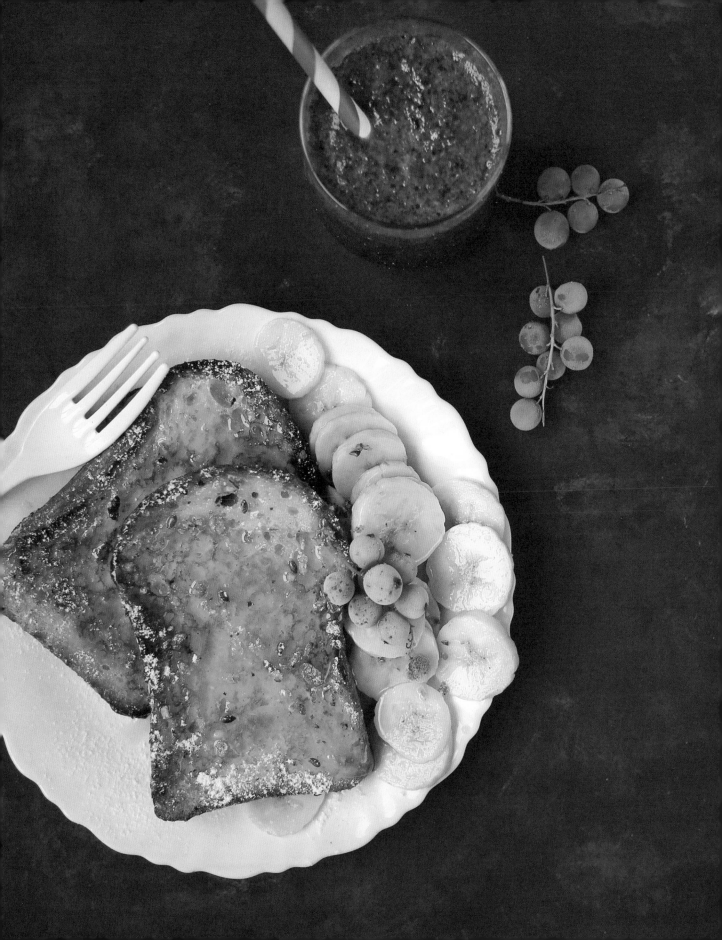

Pro-digestion
BREAKFAST
(1 pancake per pregnant woman!)

Serve the pancakes with the well-chilled smoothie.

Pancakes
WITH CHESTNUT FLOUR

MAKES 15–20 PANCAKES
PREPARATION TIME 10 MINUTES
RESTING TIME 30 MINUTES
COOKING TIME 10 MINUTES

110 g (3¾ oz) chestnut flour
2 tablespoons sugar
1 teaspoon baking powder
½ teaspoon salt
250 ml (9 fl oz/1 cup) pasteurised milk
1 free-range egg, separated
40 g (1½ oz) butter, melted
1 teaspoon liquid vanilla extract
1 knob of butter or coconut oil, for frying
a little agave syrup (or maple syrup)
a few berries, fresh or frozen
1 small handful crushed hazelnuts

Mix together the chestnut flour, sugar, baking powder
and salt in a mixing bowl. Whisk the milk and egg
yolk in a small bowl, then mix in the milk and melted
butter. In another bowl, beat the egg white with a little
salt to form firm peaks. Stir the dry mixture into the
wet mixture and, using a rubber spatula, gently fold
in the egg white. Let the batter rest for 30 minutes.

Melt a knob of butter or some coconut oil in a frying
pan. Pour in a small ladle full of batter. Cook for about
2 minutes, or until small bubbles form, then turn the
pancake over. Repeat until you have used all the batter.
Drizzle the warm pancakes with maple or agave syrup
and add a few berries and some chopped hazelnuts.

TIP: If you're short on time, you can add the egg whole
without beating the egg white.

Peach smoothie
WITH MINT + SPINACH

MAKES 2 LARGE GLASSES
PREPARATION TIME 5 MINUTES

2 peaches, in large pieces
1 sprig mint or a handful of leaves
1 handful baby spinach leaves, well washed
1 tablespoon agave syrup or flower honey

Liquidise all of the ingredients in a blender.
Add a little water to thin out the smoothie.

SUGGESTION: choose organic herbs and
fruits to keep the vitamin-packed skin.

Gluten-free recipe

A breakfast without wheat! Instead it uses chestnut flour
for super-digestible pancakes.

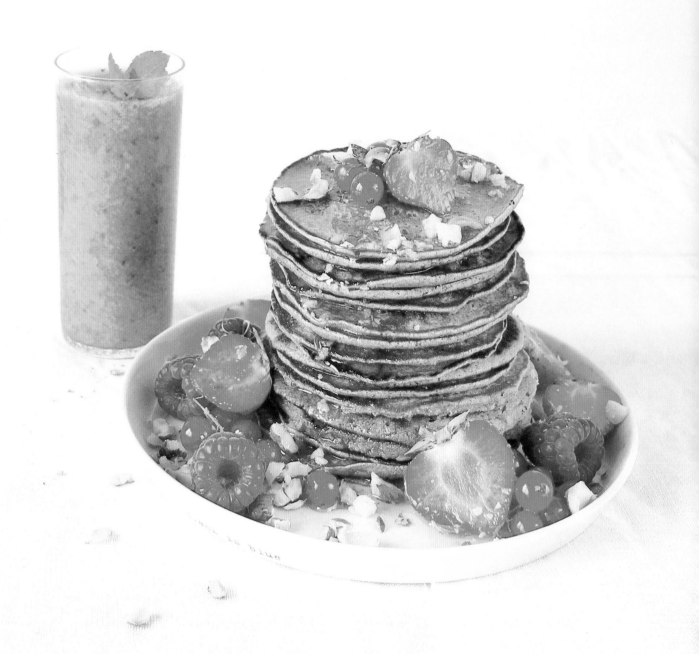

Special snack
CUPBOARD

An up-and-down appetite and small meals during the first month often leads to feeling peckish during the day. Here are a few tips to tide you over until lunch time.

Craving something sweet

There's nothing like dried fruit, nuts and seeds! They are filling and need to be chewed well, which contributes to the feeling of fullness.
- "Trail mix"-style packets of dried fruit/nuts/seeds
- Dried fruits (mango, raisins, cranberries, apricots)
- Fresh pieces of coconut

Craving something savoury

Raw vegetable sticks are good with drinks, but also as a portable snack in a zip-lock bag. Plus, raw vegetables are more easily digested as a snack when your stomach is empty and ready. For something crunchy and savoury, check packets and choose the least salty products: the difference between them is sometimes enormous. And if you have a little time, don't hesitate to go for home-made popcorn or crackers.
- Raw vegetable sticks
- Multigrain crackers
- Salted popcorn

Craving something to drink?

You should limit soft drinks, but in nine months you'll quickly become tired of orange juice. To stay hydrated and have a little variety when you're having a break, there are fresh fruit juices or smoothies, which are always better in nutritional terms than a juice in a can. For a lighter drink, this is the time to visit a fine food store and fill up on herbal teas and syrups.
- fresh fruit juices: squeezed, liquidised, juiced
- vegetable juice: tomato juice
- herbal teas in lolly (candy) flavours: mint + licorice; coconut + vanilla; apple + hibiscus + berries
- syrups or cordials: white peach syrup + lemon juice; guava syrup + mandarin syrup; strawberry syrup + melon syrup

Snacks
TO COMBAT FATIGUE

*A fresh, hydrating and thirst-quenching drink to
go with a bag of dried fruit and nut mix.*

Dried fruit + nut
SNACKS

Traditional version

In a small zip-lock bag, combine 3 tablespoons
of sultanas, 3 tablespoons of dried cranberries,
1 tablespoon of unblanched almonds and
1 tablespoon of cashew nuts.

Tropical version

In a small zip-lock bag, combine 2 tablespoons
of sultanas, 1 tablespoon of dried banana chips,
1 tablespoon of flaked coconut, 2 tablespoons
of chopped dates.

Lemon iced tea

MAKES 1 LITRE
PREPARATION TIME 10 MINUTES
RESTING TIME 30 MINUTES

Brew 1 teabag of breakfast-style black tea with
2 tablespoons of raw sugar in 1 litre (35 fl oz/4 cups)
of boiling water for 5–10 minutes. Remove the
teabag. Add 1 organic lemon, sliced, and chill
until serving.

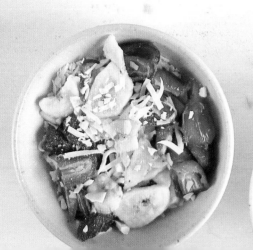

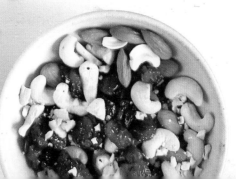

Snacks
TO AID DIGESTION

Lemon verbena with its antispasmodic properties
and stewed fruit for easy digestion.

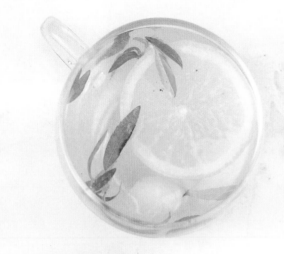

Herbal tea for digestion
WITH GINGER + LEMON

MAKES 1 TEAPOT
PREPARATION TIME 5 MINUTES

Infuse 1 cm (½ inch) piece of ginger, peeled and grated, in the juice of ½ an organic lemon and a few leaves of lemon verbena for 5 minutes.

NOTE: Also delicious in summer as an iced tea.

Light compote
APPLE + PEAR + LEMON

MAKES 2 SMALL BOWLS
PREPARATION TIME 5 MINUTES
COOKING TIME 10 MINUTES

Place 1 apple and 1 pear, peeled and diced, in a saucepan and sprinkle with the juice of ½ an organic lemon. Heat on a high heat for 10 minutes with a little water, covered. If needed, sweeten with 1 teaspoon of vanilla sugar.

VARIATION: In winter, replace the pear with ½ banana, and in summer with a well washed apricot.

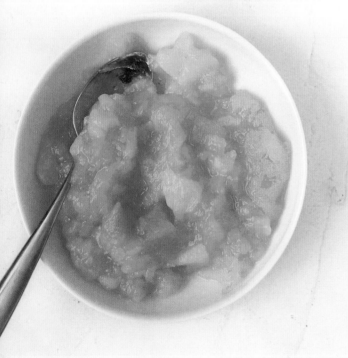

Snacks
TO COMBAT NAUSEA

A fresh fruit juice to go with little radish, cucumber and dill sandwiches, excellent for an upset stomach.

Crisp mini sandwiches
CUCUMBER + RADISH + DILL

MAKES 2 TRIANGLES
PREPARATION TIME 10 MINUTES
RESTING TIME 30 MINUTES

Slice ½ a cucumber and some radishes into thin rounds,
sprinkle with salt and let them rest for 30 minutes.
Dry them on paper towels. Spread three slices of pumpernickel
(rye) bread with your choice of spreadable cream cheese.
Lay the rounds of cucumber and radish on top, overlapping
them slightly. Add a little organic lemon juice and a turn of
the pepper mill and scatter with snipped sprigs of dill. Place
the three topped slices on top of each other and close the
sandwich with the last slice of bread. Cut into triangles.

EXTRA-SOUR VERSION: Add thin rounds of gherkin.

Apple juice
WITH FENNEL + LIME

MAKES 2 GLASSES OF JUICE
PREPARATION TIME 5 MINUTES

Juice 3 apples and ½ bulb of fennel. Add the juice
of 1 organic lime and serve immediately.

TIP: For a quick version, mix a good-quality bottled
apple juice with freshly squeezed organic lime juice.

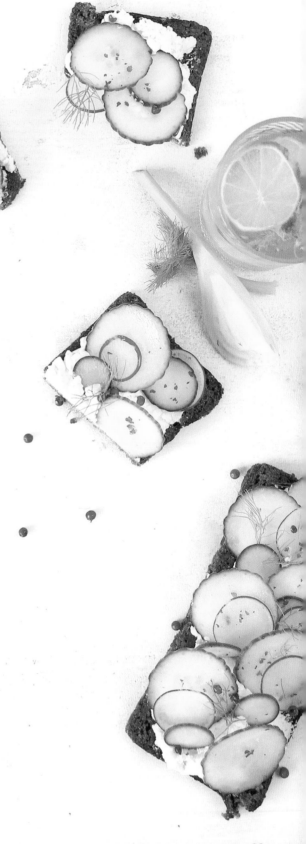

Mixed plate
No. 1
lemon chicken + couscous + avocado + radish

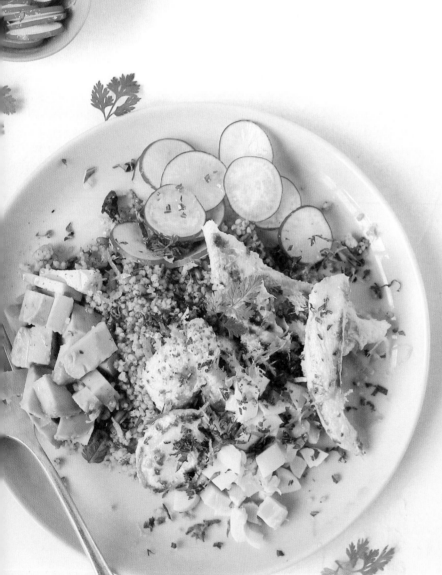

MAKES 1 PLATE
PREPARATION TIME 15 MINUTES
MARINATING TIME 10 MINUTES
COOKING TIME 10 MINUTES

80 g (2¾ oz) chicken tenderloins or 1 small
    chicken breast, sliced
2 tablespoons plain yoghurt
zest and juice of 1 small organic untreated lemon
80 g (2¾ oz) couscous or burghul (bulgur)
salt and freshly ground pepper
1 tablespoon walnut oil
½ avocado
olive oil
2 radishes, well washed and sliced into thin rounds
1 heart of palm, cut into sticks
1 sprig chervil, flat-leaf (Italian) parsley or
    chives, chopped

Combine the sliced chicken with the yoghurt, zest and
half the lemon juice. Marinate for 10 minutes. Cook
the couscous according to the instructions on the
packet. Season lightly with salt and add a little walnut
oil. Dice the avocado and lightly coat with lemon.

Heat a little olive oil in a frying pan and
brown the pieces of chicken. At the end of
the cooking time, add the marinade and cook
for a few minutes more, until piping hot.

Arrange all the ingredients on a plate and
scatter with chopped herbs. Season.

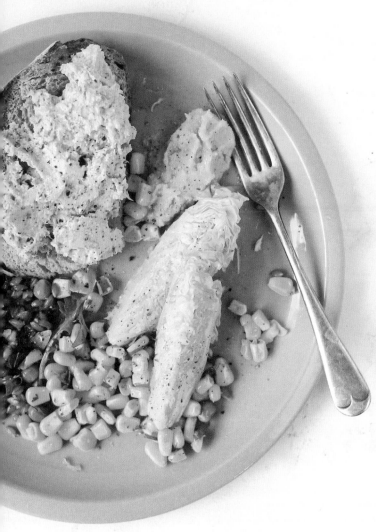

Mixed plate
No. 2
spelt with peas
+ sweet corn with coriander + tuna sandwich

MAKES 1 PLATE
PREPARATION TIME 15 MINUTES
COOKING TIME 5 MINUTES

50 g (1¾ oz) spelt (or another grain such as farro or barley)
50 ml (1¾ fl oz) olive oil (or hazelnut oil), plus extra,
    for drizzling, as required
20 g (¾ oz) peas (fresh or frozen)
1 small handful rocket (arugula), well washed
1 sprig mint, chopped
½ spring onion (scallion), peeled and thinly sliced
½ baby gem lettuce, well washed
70 g (2½ oz/½ small tin) sweet corn, drained
2 sprigs coriander (cilantro), chopped
salt and freshly ground pepper
1 teaspoon tahini (sesame paste)
juice of ½ organic lemon

Tuna sandwich
50 g (1¾ oz/½ small tin) tuna in water, drained
1 tablespoon organic lemon juice
1 teaspoon mayonnaise
1 slice wholemeal (whole-wheat) multigrain bread, toasted

Cook the spelt according to the instructions on the packet;
drain. Mix with a drizzle of olive oil and cool. Cook the peas
for 5 minutes in salted boiling water, then drain and refresh
in cold water. Combine the rocket with the mint and onion,
then add the spelt and peas. Cut the lettuce in two and
drizzle with olive oil. Mix the corn with the coriander.

For the sauce: mix the tahini with the lemon juice and the
remaining olive oil. Adjust the seasoning and whisk.

For the tuna sandwich: flake the tuna with the lemon
juice and mayonnaise. Season with salt and pepper.
Mix together well. Spread on the toasted bread. Put
together a plate with all the different elements.

TIP: Whole grains often take a long time to cook. You can
cook them in advance and store them in an airtight container
in the refrigerator for 3 days to use for quick salads during
the week.

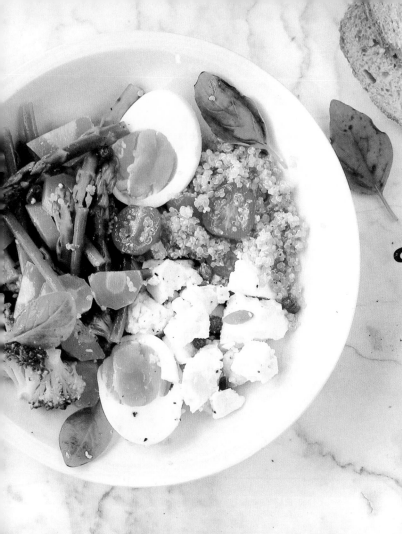

Mixed plate
No. 3
crunchy vegetables + rice + egg + ricotta sauce

Blanch all the vegetables except the tomatoes in boiling salted water for 5 minutes. Cool them down straight away in cold water so they stay nice and crisp. Cook the egg in boiling water for 9 minutes, then run it under cold water and remove the shell. Drizzle the rice with olive oil and let it cool. Combine the cherry tomatoes with the rice and the oregano.

For the sauce: mix together the ricotta, basil and capers. Thin out the mixture with a tablespoon of cold water and season.

Arrange all the ingredients on a plate, add the halved hard-boiled egg, scatter with shredded basil and serve with the bowl of ricotta sauce.

MORE SAUCES: For a more acidic sauce, add a little olive oil, a small teaspoon of honey-mustard sauce and 1 finely chopped chive.

For a vitamin-rich fish sauce, add: 1 tablespoon Vietnamese fish sauce + 1 teaspoon seaweed flakes, which are full of vitamins D, A and omega-3s.

MAKES 1 PLATE
PREPARATION TIME 10 MINUTES
COOKING TIME 20 MINUTES

½ carrot, peeled and sliced into rounds
2 spears of asparagus, well washed and cut in half
2 broccoli florets, broken up
1 handful green beans, trimmed
1 organic egg
50 g (1¾ oz) cooked brown rice or quinoa
olive oil, to drizzle
2 cherry tomatoes
1 pinch of dry or fresh oregano

Ricotta sauce
2 tablespoons ricotta
1 sprig basil, well washed and chopped
1 teaspoon capers

Mixed plate
No. 4
lemon zucchini + artichoke
+ beetroot with walnuts + lentils + avocado

MAKES 1 PLATE
PREPARATION TIME 15 MINUTES
COOKING TIME 30 MINUTES

Salad

½ zucchini (courgette)
organic lemon juice, to drizzle
olive oil, to drizzle
salt and freshly ground pepper
1 tablespoon pine nuts
1 handful peeled broad beans (fresh or frozen)
1 artichoke heart (fresh or tinned), cut into cubes
40 g (1½ oz) lentils
½ avocado, thinly sliced
½ beetroot (beet), raw, peeled and thinly sliced,
    or cooked and diced
1 handful shelled and roughly chopped walnuts
1 fresh fig, well washed, or ½ slice pineapple
    (fresh or in syrup), thinly sliced

Sauce

1 tablespoon white miso (from Asian food stores)
juice of 1 organic lemon
1 small piece of ginger, peeled and grated
1 tablespoon olive oil
½ tablespoon honey

Peel the zucchini into strips using a vegetable peeler. Heat a saucepan of water fitted with a steamer basket and bring to the boil. Steam the zucchini for 5 minutes: it should stay crisp. Cool, then drizzle with lemon juice and olive oil. Season lightly with salt and pepper and add the pine nuts.

Heat a saucepan of salted water and bring to the boil. Add the broad beans and artichoke heart and cook for 5 minutes, then drain and refresh them in cold water. Drizzle the artichoke with olive oil and salt lightly.

Cook the lentils for 20 minutes in a saucepan of salted water. Drain them and dress with olive oil. Combine the avocado with the lentils, and the beetroot with the walnuts.

For the sauce: mix the miso with the lemon juice and ginger. Add the oil and honey and whisk to emulsify. To serve, arrange all the ingredients on a plate and pour over the sauce.

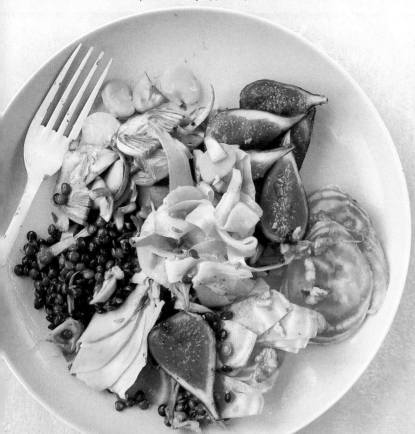

Vegan recipe

This is a 100% vegan recipe. For a perfectly balanced meal, you need fibre (lentils, walnuts, pine nuts, broad beans), a little good fat (from the avocado) and carbohydrates (figs). All served here with a miso sauce that gives a slightly malty flavour.

Fresh
AFTERNOON TEA

There's a mint tea for hydration without too much sugar and you can fill up on vitamin C and fibre with fresh fruit in every season.

Summary fruit salad
BLUEBERRIES + REDCURRANTS + APRICOTS + WATERMELON

MAKES 2 SMALL BOWLS
PREPARATION TIME 5 MINUTES – RESTING TIME 1 HOUR
5 strawberries
1 handful blueberries or blackberries
1 handful redcurrants
2 apricots
1 small slice watermelon
150 ml (5 fl oz) orange juice

Wash, peel and cut the fruit into cubes. Mix together. Add the orange juice and let it rest for 1 hour in the refrigerator.

Winter fruit salad
ORANGE + MANGO + BANANA

MAKES 2 SMALL BOWLS
PREPARATION TIME 5 MINUTES – RESTING TIME 1 HOUR
1 organic orange
½ mango
½ banana
150 ml (5 fl oz) organic orange juice
1 pomegranate, seeds extracted

Cut off the orange peel with a knife, removing the membrane at the same time, and take out the segments. Cut them in two. Dice the flesh of the mango and slice the peeled banana into rounds. Mix together. Add the orange juice and let it rest for 1 hour in the refrigerator. Scatter the pomegranate seeds over the fruit salad.

Mint tea

MAKES 1 MUG OR 2 SMALL CUPS
PREPARATION TIME 10 MINUTES
4 or 5 sprigs mint
200 ml (7 fl oz) hot water
1 sugar cube or 1 teaspoon honey

Infuse the mint leaves in hot water for 10 minutes, then remove. Add the sugar or honey and stir.

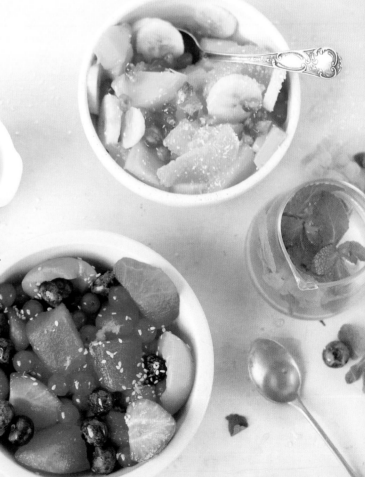

Savoury
AFTERNOON TEA

A protein-rich break during the day to keep you going comfortably until evening.

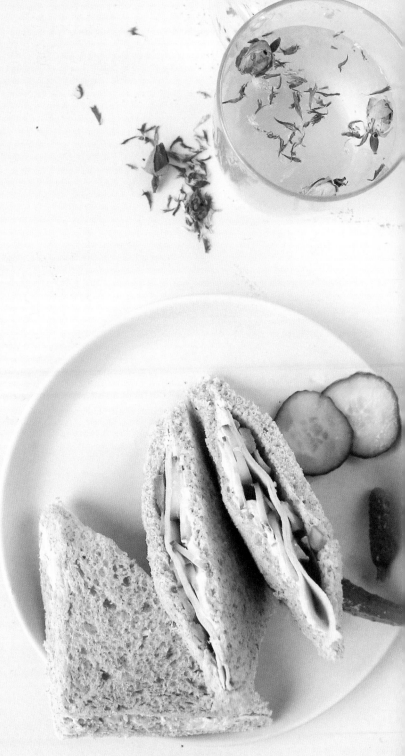

Mini turkey sandwich
WITH CUCUMBER + YOGHURT SAUCE

MAKES 1 SANDWICH
PREPARATION TIME 3 MINUTES
2 slices wholemeal (whole-wheat) sandwich bread
1 tablespoon Greek-style yoghurt
¼ cucumber, sliced into rounds
1 slice turkey ham
1 small gherkin, thinly sliced

Spread the bread with yoghurt. Lay the cucumber, turkey ham and sliced gherkin in the middle of one of the slices. Close the sandwich, press the edges firmly so the 2 slices stick together, then cut into triangles.

Rose tea

MAKES 1 MUG OR 2 SMALL CUPS
PREPARATION TIME 10 MINUTES
1 handful of rose tea mix
250 ml (9 fl oz/1 cup) hot water
honey, to taste

Infuse the rose tea in hot water for 10 minutes, then remove the flowers. Add the honey and stir.

Fried rice
WITH CASHEW NUTS
baby spinach + coriander

SERVES 2
PREPARATION TIME 15 MINUTES
COOKING TIME 15 MINUTES

100 g (3½ oz) basmati rice
3 tablespoons olive oil
  or grapeseed oil
1 pinch of salt
250 ml (9 fl oz/1 cup) water
50 g (1¾ oz) cashew nuts
1 garlic clove, peeled and crushed
½ onion, thinly sliced
1 pinch of cumin
1½ teaspoons coriander seeds
2 handfuls baby spinach leaves,
  well washed
zest of 1 organic lemon
salt and freshly ground pepper
chilli (optional)

In a deep lidded frying pan, dry toast the rice, covered, for 2–3 minutes until it smells good. Add the oil, salt and water. Let the rice cook on a low heat for about 10 minutes until the water is completely absorbed. Set the rice aside in a mixing bowl.

Return the frying pan to the heat and toast the cashew nuts, garlic, onion, cumin and coriander seeds. Stir constantly for 3–4 minutes. Add the baby spinach and cook for a few more minutes, stirring. Add the rice and mix everything together. Add the lemon zest, season generously with pepper and spike with a little chilli if you like.

TIP: This rice can also be eaten as a cold salad the next day with a little well-cooked sliced chicken, sautéed at the same time as the onion.

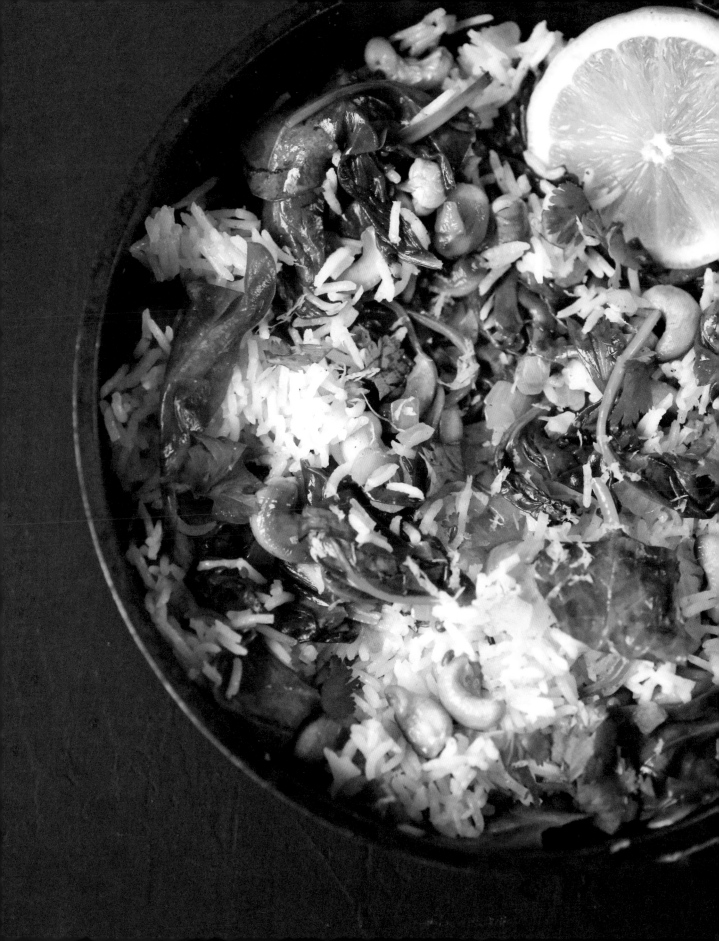

Cherry tomato
SAVOURY CLAFOUTIS
with yellow zucchini + fresh goat's cheese

MAKES 2 CLAFOUTIS
PREPARATION TIME 15 MINUTES
COOKING TIME 35 MINUTES

2 free-range eggs
3 tablespoons pasteurised milk
salt and freshly ground pepper
30 g (1 oz) fresh goat's cheese,
   crumbled
1 small yellow or green zucchini
   (courgette)
olive oil
1 garlic clove, peeled and crushed
½ bulb spring onion (scallion)
   (or yellow onion or sweet onion),
   peeled and thinly sliced
50 g (1¾ oz) cherry tomatoes
1 teaspoon raw (demerara) sugar
a few leaves of basil, well washed
   (or dried oregano)
20 g (¾ oz) grated emmental, gruyère
   or comté (French gruyère) cheese
mixed salad leaves and flat-leaf
   (Italian) parsley, well washed,
   to serve

Preheat the oven to 180°C (350°F). Butter two ramekins, 8 cm (3¼ inch) in diameter. Beat the eggs with the milk in a mixing bowl, season with salt and pepper. Add the fresh goat's cheese and mix together. Grate the zucchini like a carrot.

Pour a little olive oil in a frying pan, then add the garlic and onion. Add the cherry tomatoes, sugar and basil. Cook for 3–4 minutes on a low heat, stirring.

Divide the tomato and zucchini mixture between the ramekins and pour the egg-milk mixture on top. Sprinkle with grated cheese. Bake for about 30 minutes, until the clafoutis are golden brown. Serve the clafoutis with a mixed salad and flat-leaf parsley.

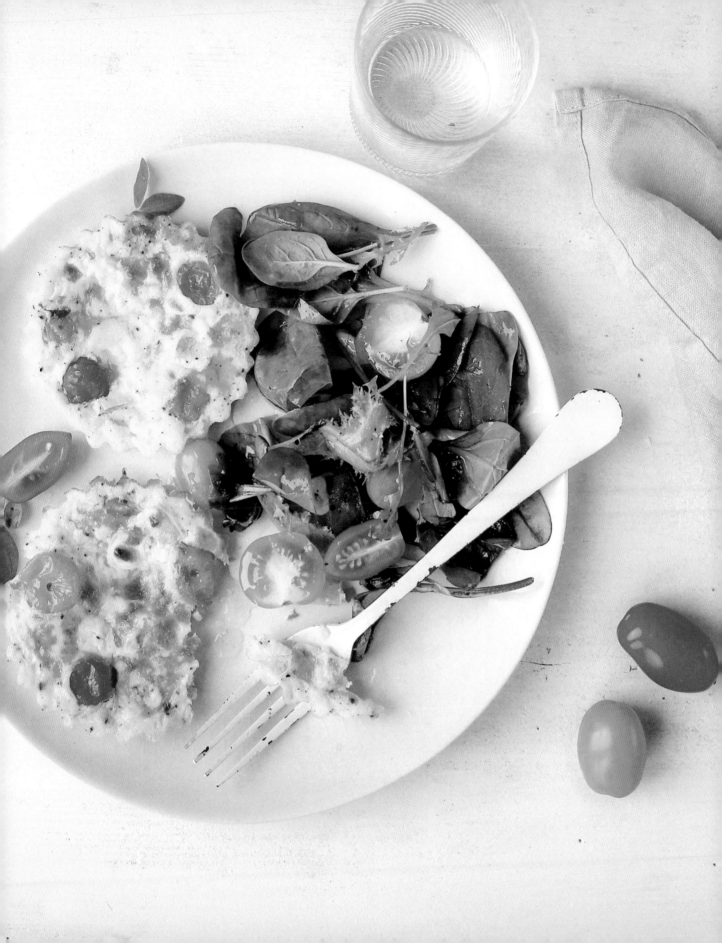

Lentil soup
WITH VEGETABLES

MAKES 2 LARGE BOWLS
PREPARATION TIME 20 MINUTES
COOKING TIME 30 MINUTES

2 tablespoons olive oil
2 sprigs fresh or dried thyme,
   plus extra, to serve
1 French shallot, peeled and sliced
1 garlic clove, peeled and crushed
1 celery stalk, chopped
1 teaspoon turmeric
1 teaspoon cumin
1 peeled tomato, roughly diced
1 generous tablespoon tomato paste
   (tomato pureé)
180 g (6½ oz) yellow or red lentils
1 large carrot, peeled and sliced
   into rounds
½ large sweet potato, cubed, or
   pumpkin (squash) (optional)
250 ml (9 fl oz/1 cup) chicken stock
250 ml (9 fl oz/1 cup) water
1 bay leaf
salt and freshly ground pepper
4–5 sprigs coriander (cilantro), well
   washed, plus extra, to serve
crème fraîche or sour cream, to serve

Heat the olive oil in a saucepan and sauté the thyme, shallot, garlic, celery, turmeric and cumin. Add the tomato and tomato paste and cook for 3 minutes. Add the lentils and carrot (and the pumpkin or sweet potato, if using), stir and cook for a few minutes.

Add the chicken stock, water, bay leaf, salt, pepper and a few sprigs of coriander. Cover the saucepan and cook for about 20 minutes: the vegetables should stay slightly al dente. Remove the thyme and bay leaf. Turn off the heat. Serve in large bowls with a little crème fraîche, coriander and thyme.

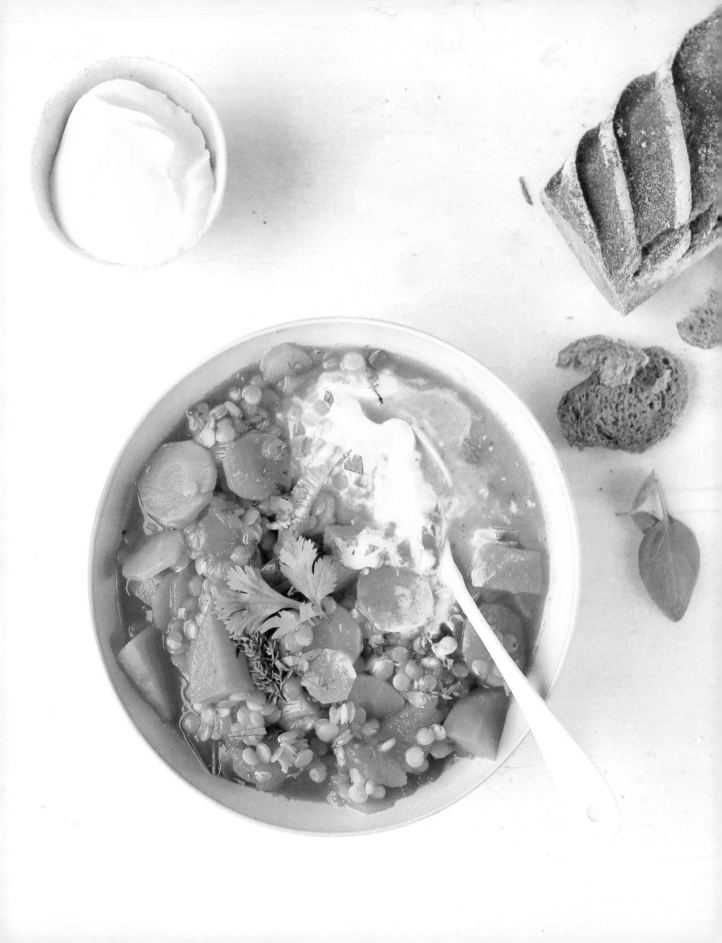

Evening
SNACKS

*If you are spreading out your meals or have had a light dinner,
don't skip an evening snack. Choose foods that
won't overload your digestive system.*

NIBBLING

Drinks

- a tea
- a glass of apple or pineapple juice
- a green tea and a glass of almond milk

Fruit, dried fruit and nuts

- a granny smith apple
- dried apricots
- a handful of raisins
- a handful of almonds

Sweet-tooth

- a square of dark chocolate with almonds
- a plain yoghurt with oatbran
- a fruit yoghurt with a small handful of granola

Crunchy

- a puffed rice cake
- crackers (multigrain, spicy, cheese, etc.)
- salted popcorn with rosemary

QUICK RECIPES

Tramezzini

Spread a thin layer of cream cheese on a slice of bread.
Place a generous spoonful of cream cheese in the
middle, top with shaved ham and a basil leaf; close with
the second slice and press the edges together to seal.
Cut into triangles.

Puffed grain cakes with toppings

Sweet:
1 puffed rice cake + 1 teaspoon of nut
butter (sesame, almond, peanut, etc.)
+ 1 teaspoon of berry jam

Savoury:
1 puffed corn cake + 1 slice swiss cheese

Mini apple sandwich

Butter 2 slices of sandwich bread very thinly.
Top one with sliced apple and a generous spoonful
of raw sugar, close with the second slice and
heat in the oven for 5 minutes. Serve warm.

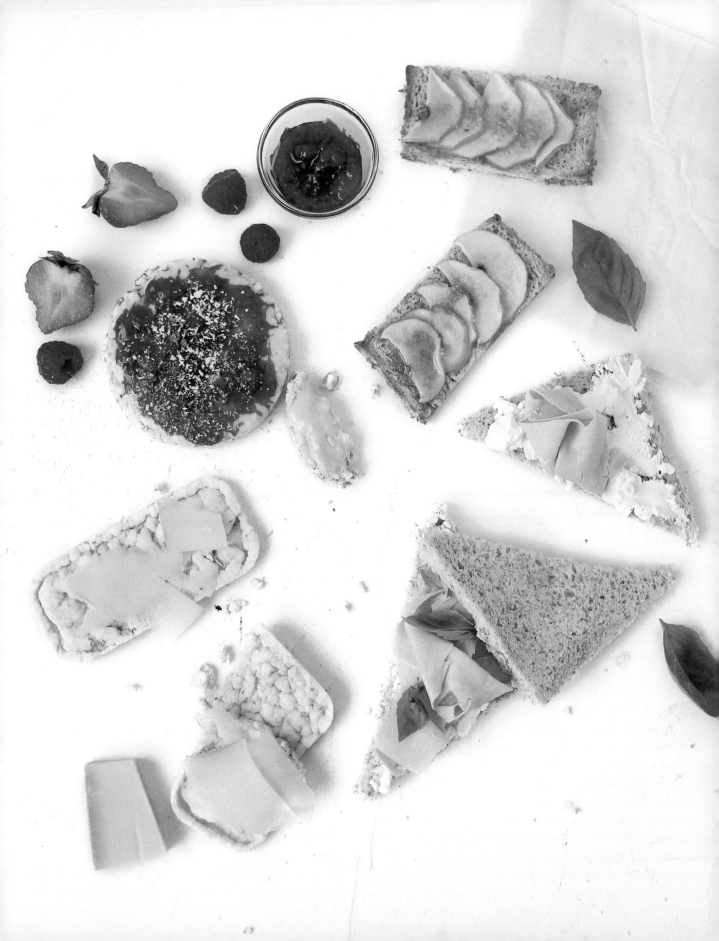

Second trimester
Eating everything

The principle: I eat everything

The nausea has passed, you have energy, you can eat everything because you're hungry, you're not too big yet, there's the joy of sharing the good news, you want to treat yourself and it's the right time to do it! You need to cook foods that will do you good and increase your energy rations. You need to fill up on calcium, fibre, vitamins and minerals, and for that it's the moment to take some time revising your shopping habits, go to the market, choose ultra fresh foods (no more ready-made meals), visit the fishmonger, the butcher, the greengrocer... When you're pregnant, you're popular with shopkeepers!

Filling ingredients

Pasta, wholemeal (whole-wheat) bread — dark rye or multigrain — for super satisfying snacks, eggs in the morning, dark chocolate for magnesium.

Calcium-rich foods

Pasteurised cheese, yoghurts, milk... but also oranges, members of the cabbage family like broccoli, tinned sardines, figs, almonds, some mineral waters.

Vitamin-rich foods

Be generous with fresh herbs, fruits such as citrus, kiwifruit and grapes, and kale. This vitamin-packed leafy green can be made into a smoothie or a juice with carrots and ginger.

Breakfast
IDEAS
(to dip into)

This is the time to fill up on antioxidant fruits, seeds and yoghurt for the calcium, and mix colours and flavours.

Craving yoghurt

For a daily dose of calcium, very important for developing the skeleton of your baby.
- Yoghurt + thyme honey + ground linseed (flaxseed) + blueberries
- Yoghurt + hazelnut butter + chocolate chips/shavings
- Yoghurt + speculaas (speculoos/Dutch spiced biscuits) (or gingerbread biscuit) + raspberries

Craving toast

Fresh fruits can replace spreads or jams for a version that's sharper, fresher and not as sweet.
- Spreadable cream cheese + mashed strawberries + honey + vanilla
- Mascarpone + berries + sugar
- ½ mashed avocado + juice of ½ organic lemon + grated apple

Craving protein

To satisfy the appetite that is growing every day!
- Crackers with herbs + cream cheese + ham
- Sandwich bread + scrambled egg + grated parmesan cheese
- Brioche + ½ small tub yoghurt + ½ mashed banana + sesame seeds

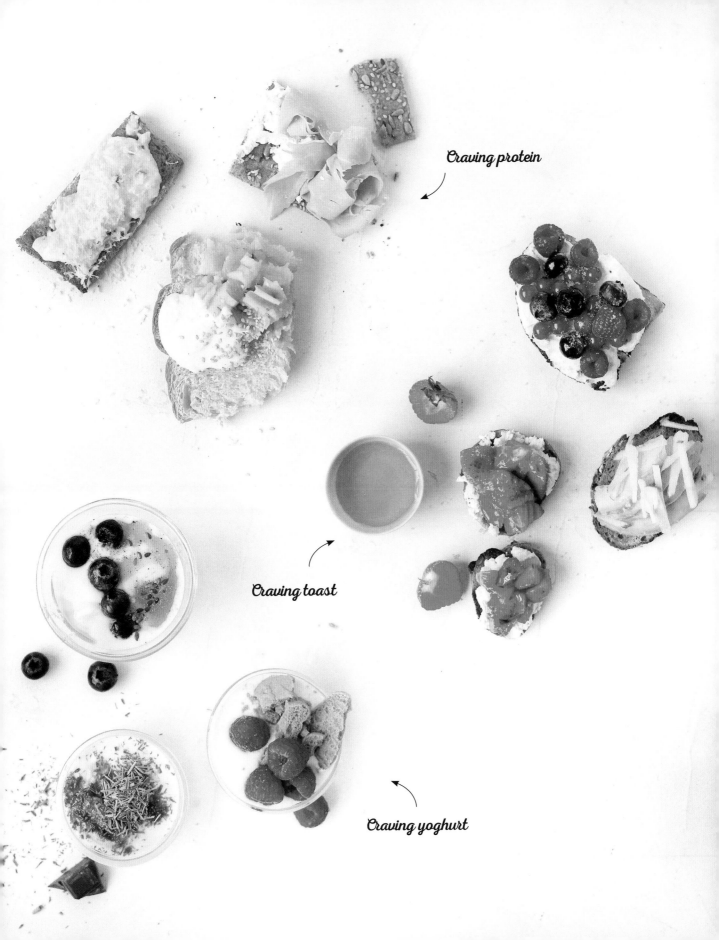

Craving protein

Craving toast

Craving yoghurt

Big appetite
BREAKFAST

*A protein-packed breakfast to fully satisfy you,
serve with a slice of good wholemeal bread.*

Baked eggs
WITH SPINACH + PARMESAN

SERVES 1 PLATE
PREPARATION TIME 10 MINUTES
COOKING TIME 15 MINUTES

1 handful baby spinach leaves, well washed
salt and freshly ground pepper
2 free-range eggs
50 g (1¾ oz) grated parmesan cheese

Preheat the oven to 200°C (400°F). Gently soften
the baby spinach in a small frying pan without adding
any fat. Season it with salt and pepper and chop
roughly with a knife. Break the eggs into a ramekin
or a cast-iron mini-frying pan. Add the parmesan and
spinach, season with pepper and bake for 10 minutes.

Cranberry juice

Antioxidant and very thirst-quenching.

Green tea with mint

Infuse a few leaves of green tea and
mint in hot water for 10 minutes.

Protein-rich breakfast

You don't always want to eat something sweet when
you wake up. A savoury breakfast is a very enjoyable
meal (rich and tasty, comforting, and lots of variety)
and full of nutrition as well. It provides a source of
energy that is low in sugar and is very filling.

Green tea with mint

Green tea contains tannins, polyphenols, vitamins and
antioxidants. It is ideal combined with mint, because
mint, which is high in vitamin C, iron and magnesium,
has digestive, antiseptic and stimulating properties. It
is recommended for pregnant women, breastfeeding
women and people with digestive problems.

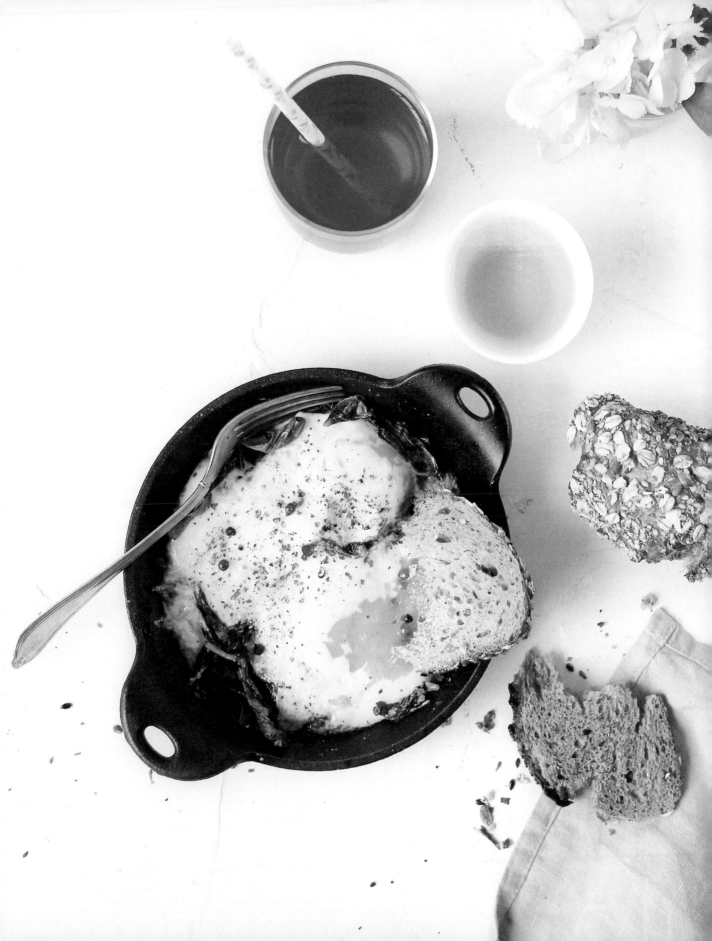

High-vitamin
BREAKFAST

A breakfast that is both filling — with the dried fruit and
nut muffins — and vitamin-charged thanks to a cocktail
with lots of the highly sought-after folic acid (vitamin B9).

Almond muffins
WITH DRIED APRICOTS

MAKES 8 MUFFINS
PREPARATION TIME 15 MINUTES
COOKING TIME 25 MINUTES

120 g (4¼ oz) flour (see note below)
10 g (¼ oz/2 teaspoons) baking powder
1 pinch of salt
60 g (1¼ oz/⅓ cup) light brown sugar
25 g (1 oz/¼ cup) flaked almonds
85 g (3 oz) soft dried apricots (about 6),
    cut into quarters
60 g (2¼ oz) butter, melted
1 egg, lightly beaten
100 ml (3½ fl oz) low-fat milk
½ teaspoon bitter almond extract (optional)

Preheat the oven to 180°C (350°F). Combine the flour,
baking powder, salt, brown sugar, flaked almonds and
dried apricots in a large mixing bowl. Place the butter,
egg, milk and extract (if using) in a smaller bowl. Pour
the wet ingredients into the dry ingredients and mix
together roughly — the batter doesn't need to be
completely smooth. Fill the holes of a buttered muffin
tray (or paper cupcake cases) two-thirds full. Bake
in the oven for 25 minutes, or until golden brown.

Carrot-orange juice
WITH GINGER + APPLE + BEETROOT
+ WATERCRESS + KALE

MAKES 2 LARGE GLASSES
PREPARATION TIME 10 MINUTES

1 handful kale or curly cabbage
2 handfuls watercress
½ raw beetroot (beet)
1 cm (½ inch) fresh ginger root,
    peeled and grated
2 carrots
2 red apples
1 handful baby spinach leaves
juice of 1 organic orange

Wash and peel all of the vegetables, then put them
through a vegetable juicer. Add the squeezed
orange juice, mix together and serve immediately.

THE NO-JUICER RECIPE

2 glasses of apple juice + 2 glasses of carrot
juice + 1 glass of squeezed orange juice + juice
of 1 lemon + 1 small piece of grated ginger

Special folic acid recipe

Folic acid plays an essential role in the production of
amino acids that promote cell growth, which makes
it important during pregnancy for the development
of the foetus. It is found in offal, legumes and dark
leafy vegetables. Try using chestnut or chickpea flour
(besan) for the muffins.

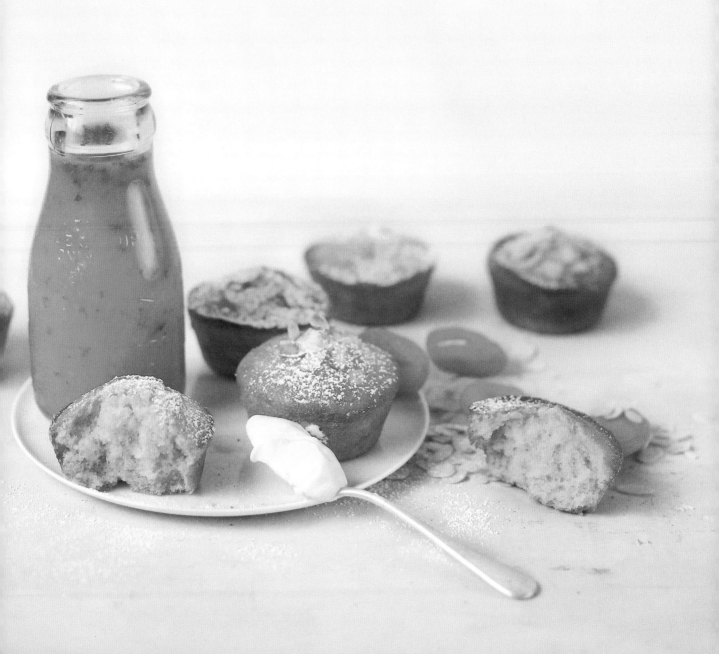

High-calcium
BREAKFAST

*A breakfast for feeling like a kid again with
a milk chocolate scone and a banana milk
to build up your calcium stores.*

Banana milk

MAKES 2 LARGE GLASSES
PREPARATION TIME 10 MINUTES

1 banana, peeled
300 ml (10½ fl oz) milk
1 teaspoon liquid vanilla extract
1 tablespoon agave syrup or sugar

Place the banana in a blender with the milk, vanilla
and agave syrup. Blend very well for 15 seconds
on maximum power and enjoy immediately.

Chocolate scones

MAKES ABOUT 10 SMALL SCONES
PREPARATION TIME 15 MINUTES
COOKING TIME 20 MINUTES

260 g (9¼ oz) flour
1 teaspoon baking powder
3 tablespoons sugar
125 g (4½ oz) chocolate chips
1 pinch of salt
75 g (2¾ oz) butter, softened (or almond butter)
1 free-range egg
3 tablespoons pasteurised milk
150 g (5½ oz) ricotta cheese (or yoghurt)
icing (confectioners') sugar

Preheat the oven to 180°C (350°F). Combine the
flour, baking powder, sugar, chocolate and salt in
a mixing bowl. Rub in the butter until the mixture
resembles breadcrumbs. In a separate bowl, whisk
the egg with the milk and ricotta. Add to the dry
mixture. Roll out the dough to a thickness of 2 cm
(¾ inch) on a well-floured surface. Cut the scones
into triangles or use a cookie cutter. Line a baking
tray with baking paper and arrange the scones on
it. Dust with icing sugar and bake for 20 minutes.

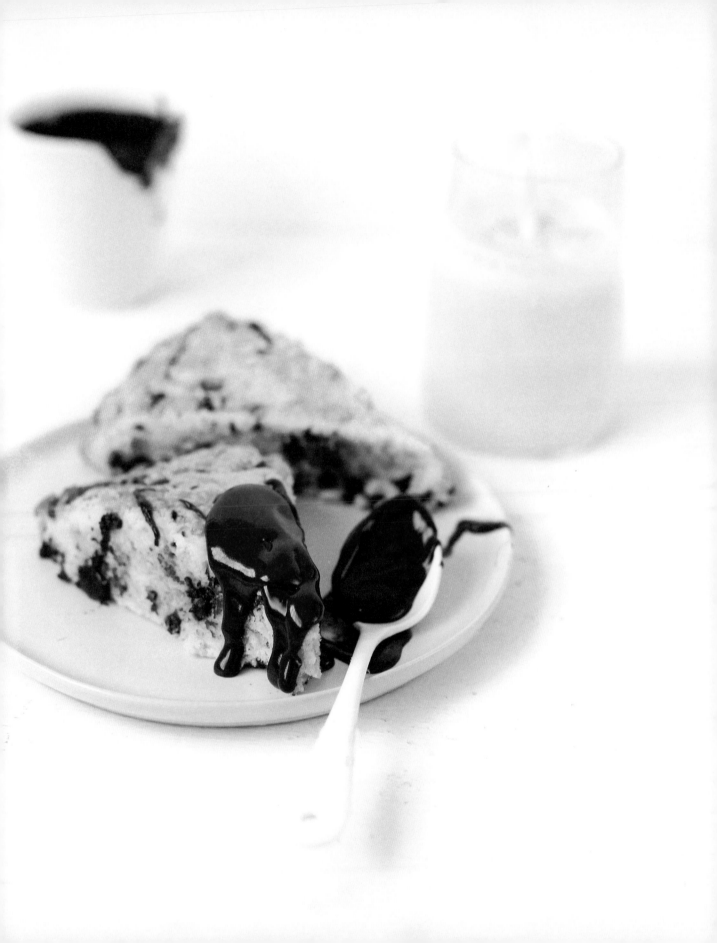

Fish cakes
WITH HERBS
and mashed potato

SERVES 2
PREPARATION TIME 30 MINUTES
COOKING TIME 15 MINUTES
+ 20 MINUTES FOR THE MASH

Fish cakes with herbs

300 g (10½ oz) white fish fillet,
    such as cod or blue-eye trevalla
1 garlic clove, peeled
1 pinch of salt
1 pinch of hot paprika
1 free-range egg white
1 teaspoon ground ginger or
    1 cm (½ inch) fresh ginger root,
    peeled and grated
4 sprigs coriander (cilantro), chopped
½ bunch chives, snipped
olive oil, for frying

Mashed potato

400 g (14 oz) potatoes, peeled
    and cut into small pieces
1 pinch of salt
200 ml (7 fl oz) low-fat milk
2 tablespoons olive oil
roughly chopped pistachio nut kernels
    (optional), to serve

For the fish cakes, process the fish fillet with the garlic, salt and paprika in a food processor to make a mince. Place this mixture in a mixing bowl. In a separate bowl, whisk the egg white with a fork, then add it to the mince. Season with salt and pepper. Add a little ground ginger and the herbs, and mix together well.

Use your hands, shape the mixture into small patties, about 6 cm (2½ inches) in diameter and not too thick (because the fish flesh needs to cook right through). Heat a little oil in a frying pan. Once it is hot, lower the heat to medium and brown the fish cakes for 2 minutes on each side.

For the mash: cook the potatoes in a large saucepan of boiling salted water for 20 minutes, then drain. Mash the potatoes with the milk and olive oil using a stick (hand-held) blender. Scatter with pistachios.

Serve the fish cakes with the mash.

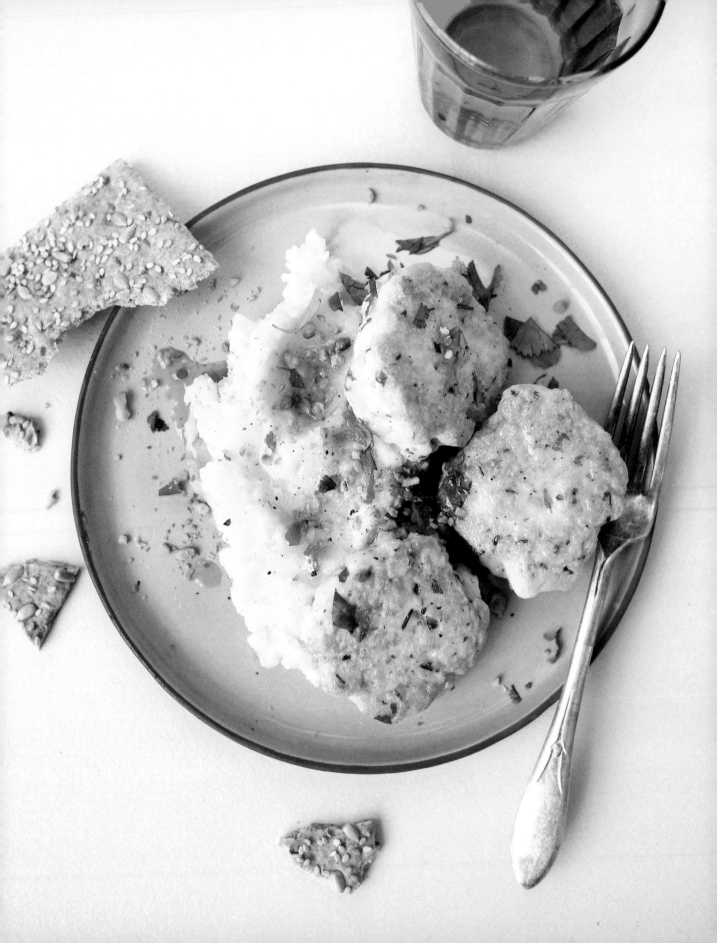

Salmon
TERIYAKI
with roasted sweet potatoes

SERVES 2
PREPARATION TIME 30 MINUTES
COOKING TIME 35 MINUTES
RESTING TIME 30 MINUTES

Salmon teriyaki

1 tablespoon organic lemon juice
1 tablespoon soy sauce
½ teaspoon raw sugar
1 teaspoon grated ginger
1–2 sprigs Thai basil (or chives or
    parsley), chopped
2 salmon fillets
1 tablespoon cornflour (cornstarch)
freshly ground pepper

Roasted sweet potatoes

2 tablespoons maple syrup
1 tablespoon mustard
2 tablespoons olive oil
salt and freshly ground pepper
2 sweet potatoes, peeled and
    cut into chips or large cubes
2 large sprigs thyme (or rosemary
    or oregano)

For the grilled salmon: mix together the lemon juice, soy sauce, sugar, ginger and Thai basil in a bowl. Make two or three cuts in the salmon fillets. Place them in a deep plate and pour over the marinade. Let them rest in the refrigerator for 30 minutes.

For the sweet potatoes: mix together the maple syrup, mustard and olive oil in a bowl. Add the sea salt and pepper. Preheat the oven to 220°C (425°F). Place the sweet potatoes in a mixing bowl, pour over the maple syrup mixture and combine to coat all of the pieces well. Arrange them on a baking tray lined with baking paper (or an oiled baking dish or tin), scatter with thyme and bake for about 25 minutes: the sweet potatoes should be well-browned and roasted.

Drain the salmon fillets and wipe them dry with paper towel. Set the fish marinade aside. Season the salmon with pepper and cook it on a hotplate or in a frying pan over high heat for 3–4 minutes on each side. Pour the marinade into a saucepan and reduce it by half. In a cup, blend the cornflour with 1 tablespoon cold water. Stir this mixture into the marinade to make a syrupy sauce. Adjust the seasoning.

Serve the fish with its sauce and the roasted sweet potatoes on the side.

VARIATION: Replace the sweet potatoes with parsnips or carrots or a mixture of each. The salmon can be replaced with tuna or a white-fleshed fish.

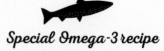

Special Omega-3 recipe

Salmon is high in good fats (omega-3s), protein, vitamins and minerals, so it is good for reducing the risk of cardiovascular diseases. It is recommended to eat oily fish such as salmon, mackerel or sardines twice a week.
Note: wild salmon contains the same amount of mercury as farmed salmon, but much fewer pesticides and less fat than non-organically farmed salmon.

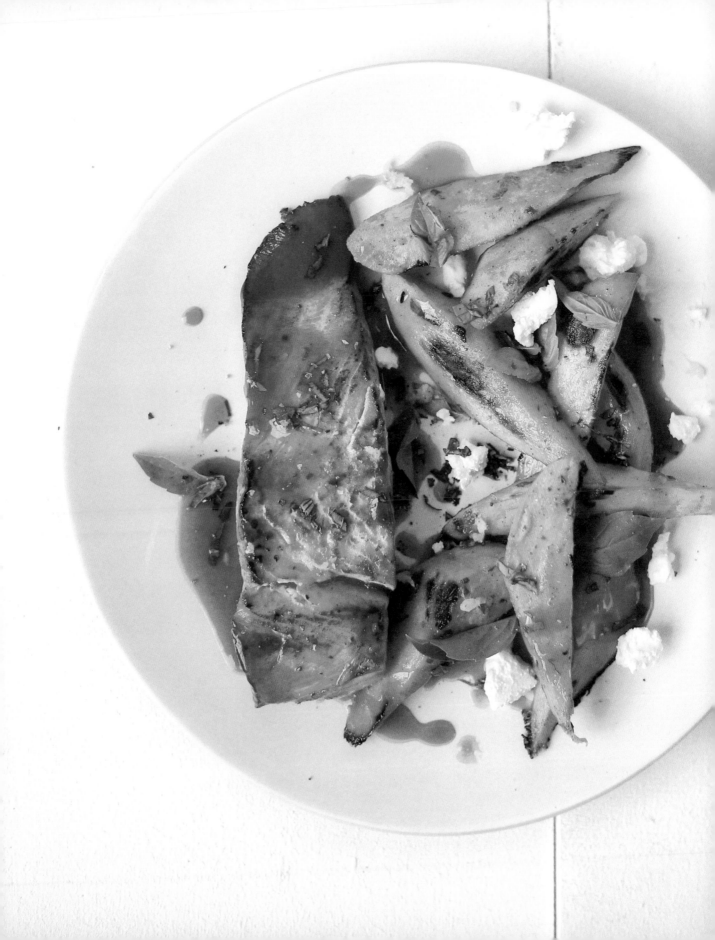

Chicken pita
WITH GRILLED CAPSICUM
tomato + cucumber + carrot + yoghurt

SERVES 2
PREPARATION TIME 20 MINUTES
COOKING TIME 20 MINUTES

1 red capsicum (pepper), seeded
olive oil, as required
2 chicken breasts, thinly sliced
1 teaspoon turmeric
1 teaspoon mild chilli powder
    (or tandoori masala)
1 teaspoon cumin
2 pita breads
1 tomato, sliced into rounds
½ cucumber, sliced into rounds
1 carrot, peeled and grated

Yoghurt sauce
125 g (4½ oz/1 small tub) plain
    yoghurt
½ teaspoon mustard or honey-
    mustard style sauce
fresh chopped herbs (chives,
    flat-leaf [Italian] parsley, dill)
1 white onion, peeled and chopped
salt and freshly ground pepper

Preheat the oven to 200°C (400°F). Roast the capsicum in the oven for about 20 minutes. When the skin blisters, take it out and place it in a plastic bag. After 2 minutes, remove from the bag and peel off the skin with the tip of a knife. Slice the capsicum into thin strips. Place it in a dish and sprinkle with olive oil.

Sauté the chicken in olive oil in a hot frying pan. Add the turmeric, mild chilli powder and ground cumin. Stir until the chicken is golden and cooked through. Season.

Cut the pita breads in half horizontally and heat them quickly in a toaster.

For the yoghurt sauce: mix together the plain yoghurt with the mustard, herbs and white onion in a bowl. Season with salt and pepper.

Put some yoghurt sauce, slices of chicken and grilled capsicum, tomato, cucumber and grated carrot in each pita bread.

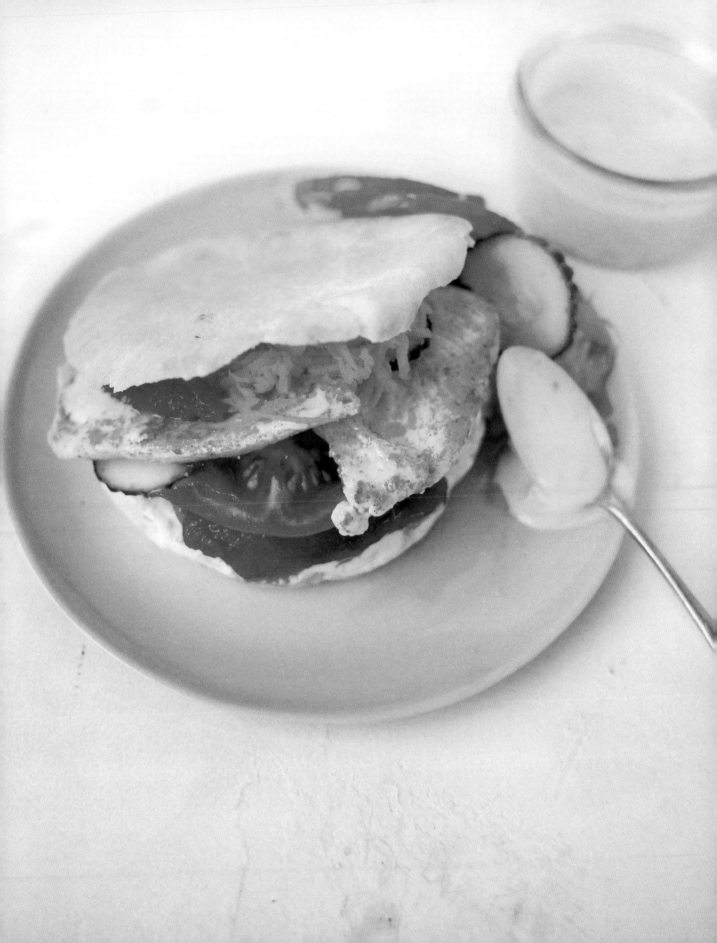

Express
SOUP WITH PESTO
beans + zucchini + pasta

SERVES 2
PREPARATION TIME 20 MINUTES
COOKING TIME 50 MINUTES

Soup

2 potatoes, peeled and diced
1 onion, peeled and thinly sliced
olive oil, as required
salt
½ zucchini (courgette), diced
100 g (3½ oz) fresh green beans,
   trimmed (or frozen if you don't
   have fresh)
3–4 basil leaves
1 large tomato, peeled and diced
100 g (3½ oz) tinned cannellini beans
100 g (3½ oz) tinned kidney beans,
   drained
80 g (2¾ oz) small soup pasta
   (pastina)

Express pesto

4–5 sprigs fresh basil
4 garlic cloves, peeled
100 g (3½ oz/1 cup) parmesan
   cheese, coarsely grated
olive oil, as required

For the soup: cook the diced potato for about 15 minutes in a large quantity of boiling water. Drain. Meanwhile, sauté the onion in a hot frying pan with some olive oil. In another saucepan, bring a little salted water to the boil and add the zucchini and green beans with a little olive oil and a few basil leaves. Cook for about 20 minutes. Add the tomato, onion, potatoes and the cannellini and kidney beans, mix together and cook for a further 10 minutes. Add the pasta and cook for another 10 minutes. Turn off the heat.

For the pesto: blend the basil leaves in a food processor with the garlic cloves, parmesan cheese and enough olive oil to make a sauce.

To serve, pour the pesto sauce over the vegetable soup.

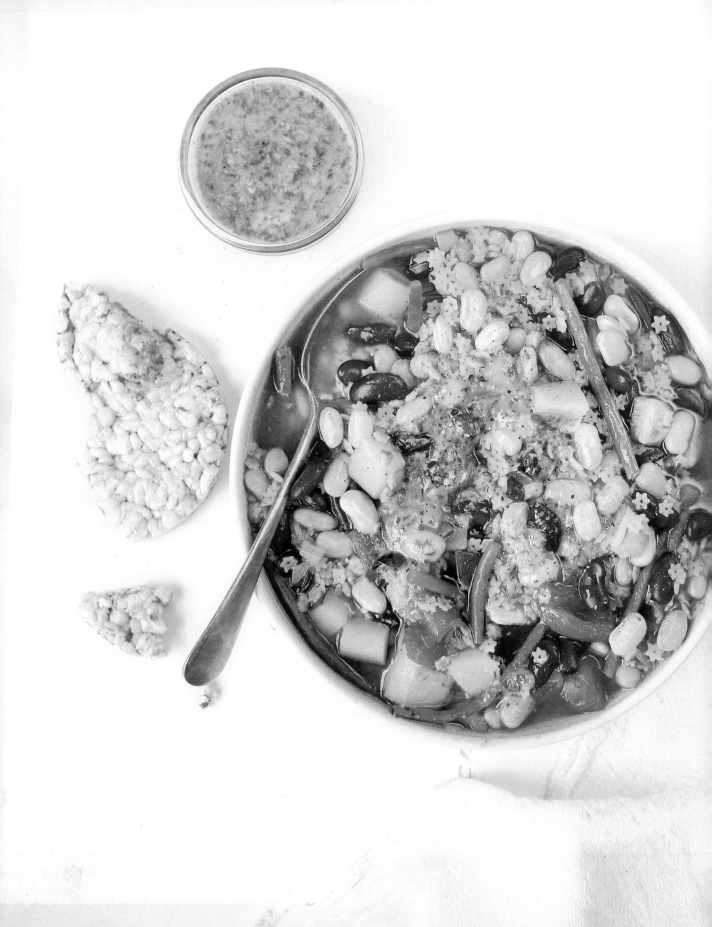

Smoked haddock
SALAD
kale + red cabbage + orange

SERVES 2
PREPARATION TIME 20 MINUTES
COOKING TIME 10 MINUTES

Salad

1 small bunch organic kale,
   stems removed
4 tablespoons olive oil
2 tablespoons sherry vinegar
salt and pepper
½ red cabbage, thinly sliced
4 raw beetroot (beets) (2 red and
   2 yellow), peeled and thinly sliced
1 organic orange, peeled into
   segments
1 handful toasted pecans
1 handful toasted pumpkin seeds
   (pepitas)

Poached haddock

500 ml (17 fl oz/2 cups) milk
200 ml (7 fl oz) water
300 g (10½ oz) smoked haddock
   fillet, or substitute hot-smoked trout,
   skinned and boned
1 teaspoon of your choice of spices
   (e.g. cloves, turmeric, aniseed, dill,
   star anise, fennel)

For the salad: clean the kale leaves and remove the centre ribs, keeping the more tender part. Mix together the oil, vinegar, salt and pepper. Massage the kale with this dressing to soften the leaves. Add the rest of the ingredients and mix together.

For the smoked haddock: heat the milk and water in a saucepan. When the liquid comes to a gentle simmer, add the fish and spices and poach for 10 minutes. Drain the haddock and flake it before serving with the salad.

Super food recipe

Kale is a super cabbage with magical properties, the new friend of the food-as-medicine movement. It is packed with antioxidants, fibre, protein and vitamins C and K. It is green and curly and a little tough-looking, but once it is dressed with olive oil or blended in a smoothie, it is delicious.

For even more super food: add antioxidant-rich pomegranate seeds.

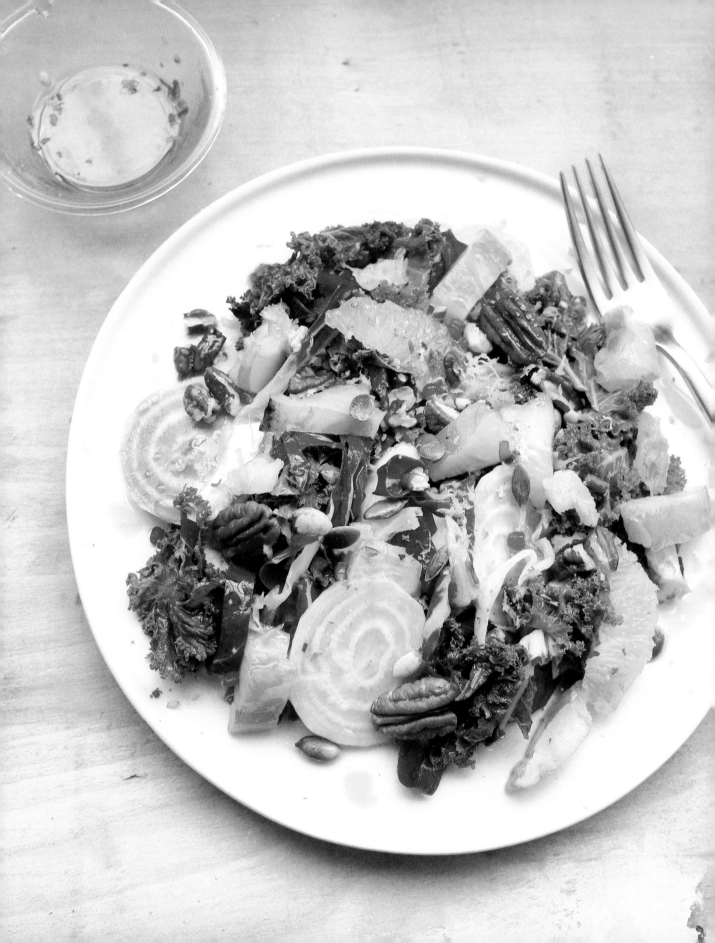

Shepherd's pie
WITH SPINACH
lamb + potatoes + jerusalem artichokes

SERVES 6
PREPARATION TIME 15 MINUTES
COOKING TIME 50 MINUTES

300 g (10½ oz) Jerusalem artichokes,
  peeled and diced
300 g (10½ oz) potatoes,
  peeled and diced
300 g (10½ oz) spinach, cooked
  and drained (or frozen spinach)
2 tablespoons crème fraîche or
  sour cream
salt and pepper
500 g (1 lb 2 oz) lamb (e.g. shoulder),
  cut into cubes
½ small bunch mint
olive oil, for frying
1 tablespoon breadcrumbs
1 tablespoon grated parmesan cheese

Preheat the oven to 180°C (350°F). Cook the Jerusalem artichokes and potatoes in a large volume of boiling salted water for about 20 minutes. Drain. Mash the spinach with a fork. Mash the artichokes and potatoes with a hand-held potato masher. Add the crème fraîche. Season with salt and pepper.

Mince the diced lamb in a food processor. Add a dozen mint leaves and process again. Season. Pour a little olive oil in a frying pan, add the lamb and sauté for 5–10 minutes, stirring often.

Spread the lamb in the base of a gratin dish or tin. Scatter with mint leaves, top with the Jerusalem artichoke and potato mash, then the spinach. Cover with breadcrumbs and parmesan. Bake for 20–25 minutes.

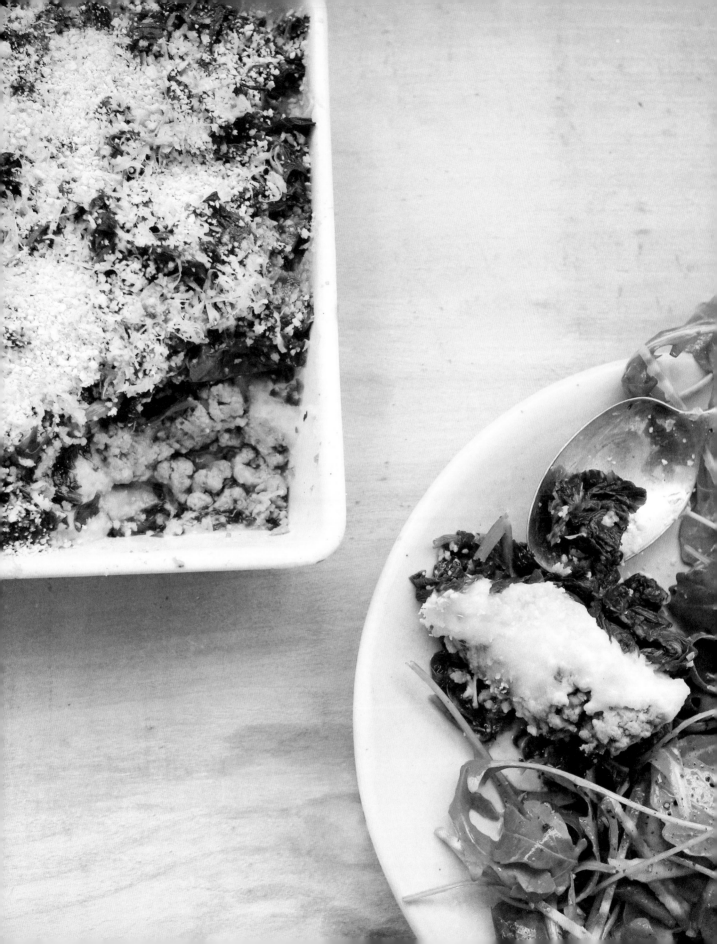

Third trimester
Eating light

The principle

The last part of pregnancy isn't the easiest: it's difficult to move around easily and your digestive system is under pressure because the baby is growing every day. The stress about the birth starts, insomnia, lower back pain, water retention… but this is no time to crumble! Don't fall back into snacking, you need to keep eating well. The baby is nourished by everything you eat and gets used to the foods that are transmitted through the amniotic fluid. Home stretch!

Foods to aid digestion

Increase fibre: lentils, cannellini beans, peas, broad beans, cabbage, wholemeal (whole-wheat) bread, prunes. Drink lots of water with lemon or mint leaves. Take advantage of peaches in summer, or else eat plums or apples and dates.

Foods to give you energy

Grains, dried fruit and nuts, fruit juice diluted with a little water (I often mix a half-glass of apple juice with a little soda water). Eat pasta or brown rice with cashews or any sort of nut!

Foods to combat stress

Magnesium-rich foods: chocolate, dried legumes, dried fruit and nuts, Brazil nuts, pepitas (pumpkin seeds), sunflower seeds, unblanched almonds, sea salt, coriander seeds.

Iron-rich foods

Black pudding, red meat, white meat, fish and eggs. Also lentils, cabbage, watercress, ginger, cinnamon and cumin seeds.

Omega-3-rich foods

Salmon, sardines, mackerel, walnuts and walnut oil, canola oil, hempseed oil, chia seeds.

Breakfast
IDEAS
(take your pick)

In the third trimester, focus on fibre and energy and give yourself little morale-boosting treats. Here are a few ideas if you want a quick and healthy breakfast.

Craving hot milk

As a change from a hot chocolate, which can be too heavy and sweet, try almond or rice milk. They are more digestible than cow's milk but just as creamy. Rice milk is high in silica for boosting calcium; almond milk is rich and delicious, it contains vitamins (A, B and E), calcium, magnesium and iron. These milks can be flavoured like ordinary milk (gently heat the milk and dissolve the flavouring in it).

• rice milk + squares of chocolate + agave syrup
• almond milk + cardamom + sugar
• cow's milk + vanilla + cinnamon +
  a few drops of caramel sauce.

Craving a quick muesli

No time to toast nuts and grains but really craving a good muesli? Here are a few combinations to try for a full load of protein, carbohydrates and fibre.

• rolled oats + pepitas (pumpkin seeds)
  + hazelnuts + grapes
• puffed quinoa + flaked coconut + dried
  mango + roughly chopped Brazil nuts
• corn flakes + sesame seeds + roughly
  chopped macadamia nuts + honey.

Craving fruit

Fruit you eat with a spoon is quick and full of vitamins.
• ½ grapefruit + raw (demerara) sugar
• 1 kiwifruit + mint
• ½ small melon + raspberry coulis.

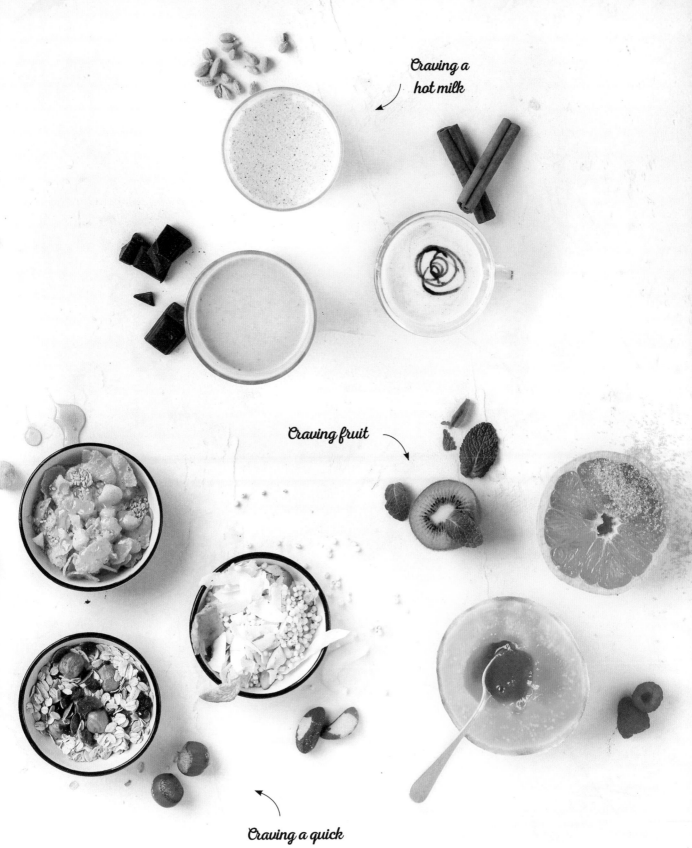

Craving a
hot milk

Craving fruit

Craving a quick
muesli

Special fibre
BREAKFAST

Whole and fibre-rich foods to regulate
your digestive system.

Green smoothie
FENNEL + GREEN APPLE + MINT

MAKES 2 LARGE GLASSES
PREPARATION TIME 10 MINUTES

½ fennel bulb
2 green apples
10 mint leaves
150 ml (5 fl oz) water
1 tablespoon agave syrup

Blend the fennel with the green apples, mint, water and
agave syrup until you have a semi-thick consistency
(about 30–45 seconds). Serve immediately.

Pear bruschetta
WITH ALMOND BUTTER + SEEDS

MAKES 2 GENEROUS BRUSCHETTA
PREPARATION TIME 10 MINUTES

2 slices rye bread
2 teaspoons unblanched almond butter
1 pear, peeled and thinly sliced
1 tablespoon linseeds (flaxseeds)
a drizzle of agave syrup (or honey)

Toast the slices of bread and spread them
with almond butter. Cover with slices of pear
and linseeds. Drizzle with a little agave syrup
and put under the grill for a moment.

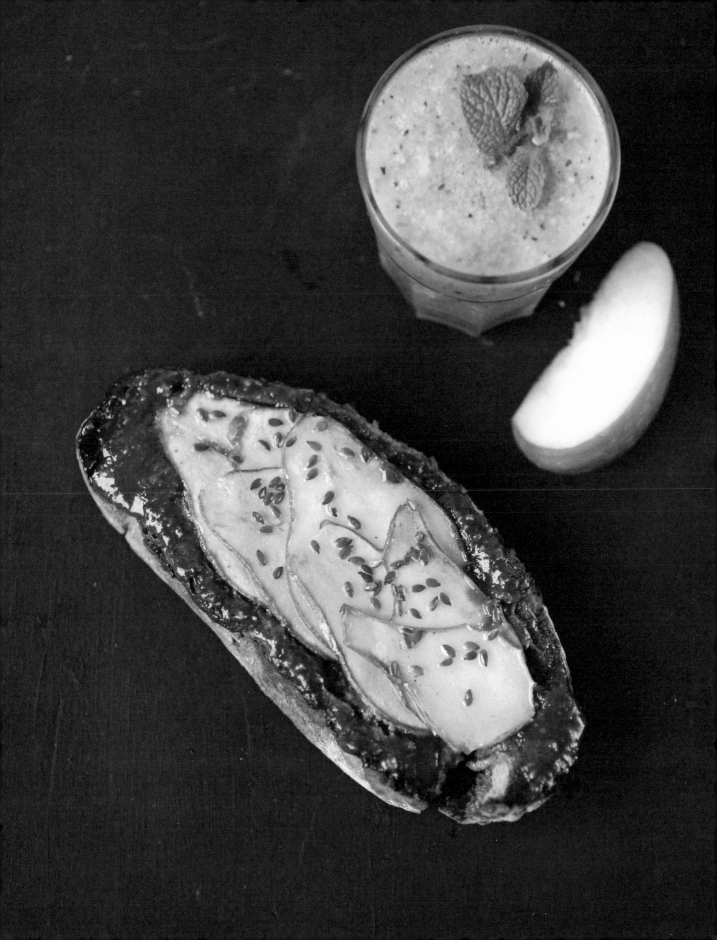

Comforting
BREAKFAST

Quick, simple, balanced.

Almond porridge
WITH ALMOND MILK + RASPBERRIES

MAKES 2 BOWLS
PREPARATION TIME 10 MINUTES

60 g (2¼ oz) rolled oats
150 ml (5 fl oz) rice or almond milk
1 tablespoon agave syrup (or honey, or maple syrup)
1 teaspoon unblanched or blanched almond butter
1 tablespoon almonds
fresh or frozen raspberries (or 1 tablespoon
   raspberry coulis)

Place the rolled oats in a saucepan with the milk
and heat for 3 minutes. Once the mixture has
thickened, add the syrup and almond butter. Mix
well and serve with the almonds, raspberries or
coulis, accompanied by a fresh orange juice.

VARIATION: You can replace the raspberries with figs
and the almonds with pepitas (pumpkin seeds) and
linseeds (flaxseeds).

Orange juice drink

MAKES 2 GLASSES
PREPARATION TIME 3 MINUTES

Squeeze 5 well-chilled organic oranges. Mix in a
shaker or briefly blend the juice in a food processor
with 100 ml (3½ fl oz) milk and serve immediately.

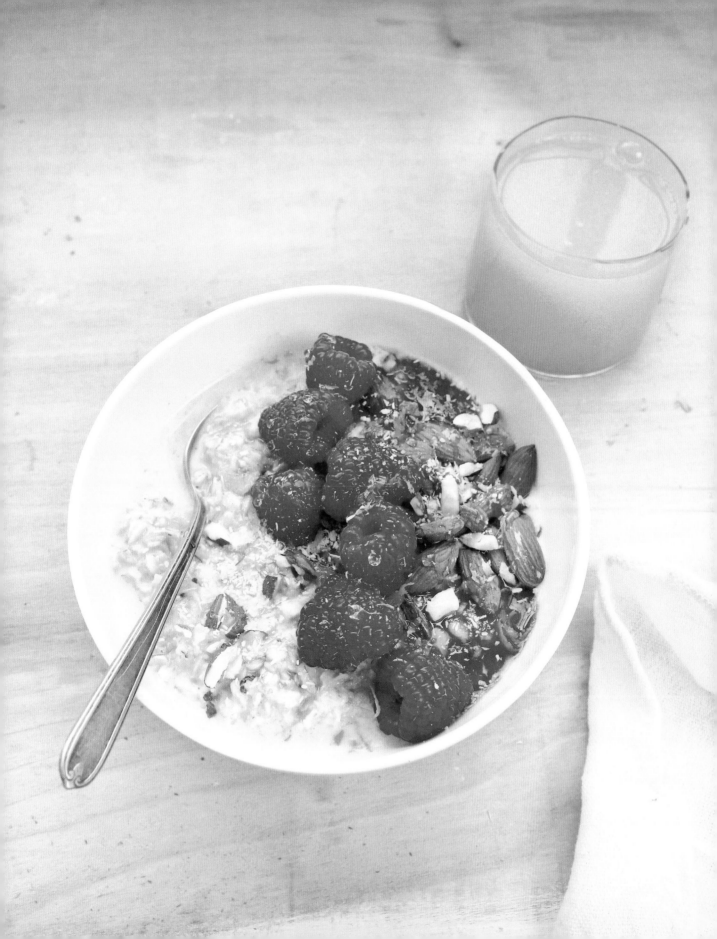

High-protein
BREAKFAST

Protein, antioxidants, calcium.

Sweet omelette
LEMON + BLUEBERRIES + POPPY SEEDS + FRUIT YOGHURT

SERVES 2
PREPARATION TIME 10 MINUTES
COOKING TIME 5 MINUTES

2 free-range eggs
1 pinch of salt
1 teaspoon maple syrup (or honey, or agave syrup)
zest of ½ organic lemon
1 teaspoon poppy seeds
1 teaspoon coconut oil (or olive oil), for frying
60 g (2¼ oz/½ small tub) yoghurt, plain or
   fruit-flavoured
1 handful fresh blueberries

Whisk the eggs in a bowl until they are very
frothy. Add the salt, syrup, lemon zest (keep
some aside) and half the poppy seeds.

Heat the coconut oil in a small frying pan and
make sure it coats the whole base of the pan.
Cook the omelette for 3 minutes on a medium
heat, then turn over and cook for another minute.
Serve the omelette with yoghurt, blueberries,
the rest of the zest and poppy seeds.

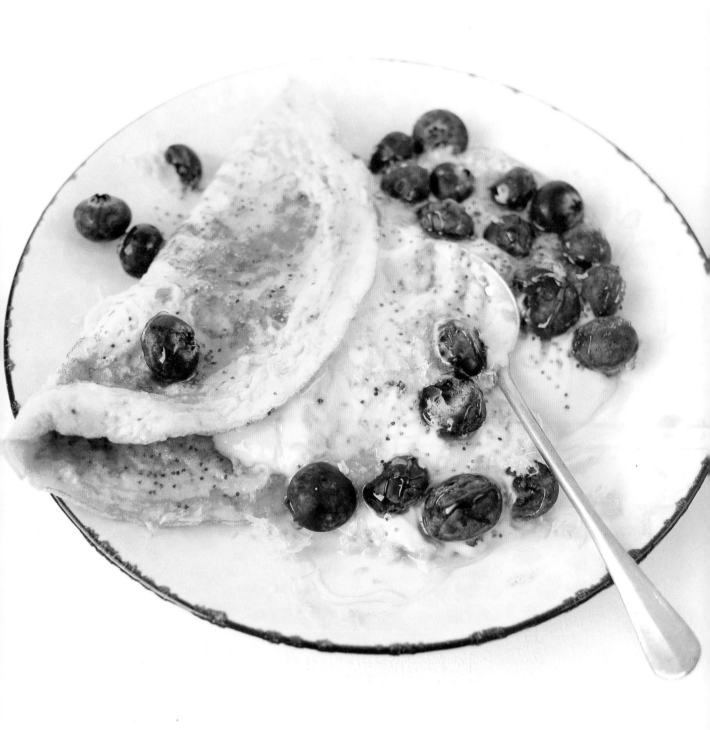

Thai beef salad
EXPRESS BÚN BÒ STYLE
beef + cucumber + peanuts

SERVES 2
PREPARATION TIME 20 MINUTES
COOKING TIME 10 MINUTES
RESTING TIME 30 MINUTES

100 g (3½ oz) thin rice noodles
500 ml (17 fl oz/2 cups) boiling water
240 g (9 oz) beef fillet steak
3 tablespoons organic lime juice
4 tablespoons Vietnamese fish sauce
2 tablespoons rice vinegar
170 ml (5½ fl oz/⅔ cup) hot water
2 tablespoons light brown sugar
1 garlic clove, peeled and sliced
1 French shallot, peeled and sliced
1 large bunch of herbs: mint, coriander
   (cilantro), Thai basil (or flat-leaf
   [Italian] parsley, or traditional basil)
1 lemongrass stem, thinly sliced
   (or lime zest)
¼ cucumber, sliced into rounds
1 carrot, peeled and grated
1 baby gem lettuce, washed
   and shredded
1 handful peanuts, roughly chopped

Place the rice noodles in a large bowl and add the boiling water. Let them soften for 8 minutes, then drain under cold water.

Grill the beef in a dry frying pan for 3 minutes on each side: it should stay pink in the middle. Let it cool on a plate. Alternatively, brush with olive oil and cook in the oven for 10 minutes at 200°C (400°F).

Thinly slice the beef. Put the lime juice, fish sauce, vinegar, hot water and sugar in a bowl. Mix together. Add the garlic, shallot, herbs, lemongrass, noodles and sliced beef. Mix together well. Add the cucumber, carrot and lettuce. Rest for 30 minutes in the refrigerator. Scatter with peanuts at serving time.

NOTE: The beef needs to be cooked to medium if you do not have immunity to toxoplasmosis (see page 9). Choose a quality piece that will stay nice and tender.

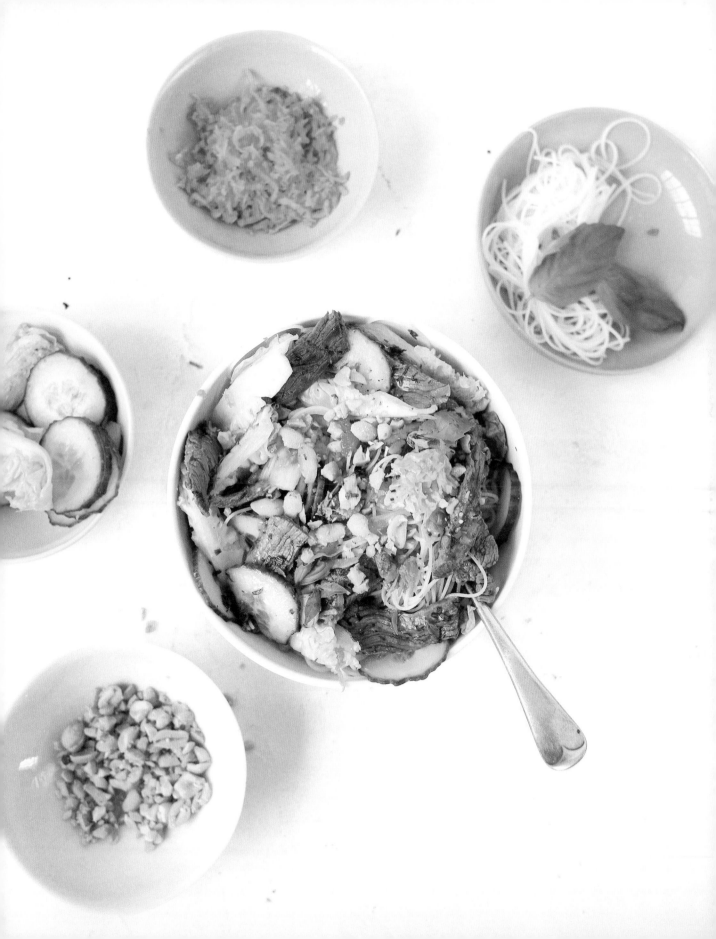

Black pudding
GRATIN
with celeriac mash

SERVES 2
PREPARATION TIME 20 MINUTES
COOKING TIME 50 MINUTES

Potato and celeriac mash

½ celeriac, peeled and cut into
   large dice
2 potatoes, peeled and cut into
   large dice
salt and freshly ground pepper
pinch of nutmeg
20 g (¾ oz) butter or 1 tablespoon
   olive oil
crème fraîche or sour cream (optional)

Black pudding with apples

200 g (7 oz) apples (e.g. golden
   delicious or gala), peeled, cut into
   large dice
1 onion, peeled and thinly sliced
pinch of nutmeg
freshly ground pepper
150 g (5½ oz) black pudding
   (blood sausage)
1 tablespoon olive oil
50 g (1¾ oz) grated cheese (such
   as gruyère or swiss cheese)

Put the diced celeriac and potatoes in a saucepan and cover with water. Bring to the boil and cook for about 15 minutes. Once the vegetables are tender, drain and mash with a potato masher. Add the salt, pepper, nutmeg and butter or olive oil.

For a creamy mash, add a spoonful of crème fraîche.

Cook the diced apples in a saucepan with a tablespoon of water for about 15 minutes. Stew the fruit gently, keeping the pieces intact.

Gently sauté the onion in a frying pan with a little olive oil. Sprinkle with nutmeg and season with pepper. Remove the skin from the black pudding and crumble it into the onion. Cook well, stirring, for 5–8 minutes.

Heat the oven grill. Alternate layers in a small baking dish or tin: potato-celeriac mash, stewed apple, black pudding, then more mash and apple. Scatter with grated cheese and brown under the grill for 15 minutes.

Iron-rich recipe

Black pudding is the champion! With 22 mg iron per 100 g (3½ oz), it represents 160% of the recommended daily intake. This is not surprising, as black pudding is made from pig's blood and iron is the main component of red blood cells. Plus, this iron is absorbed five to ten times better than the iron in vegetables or eggs.

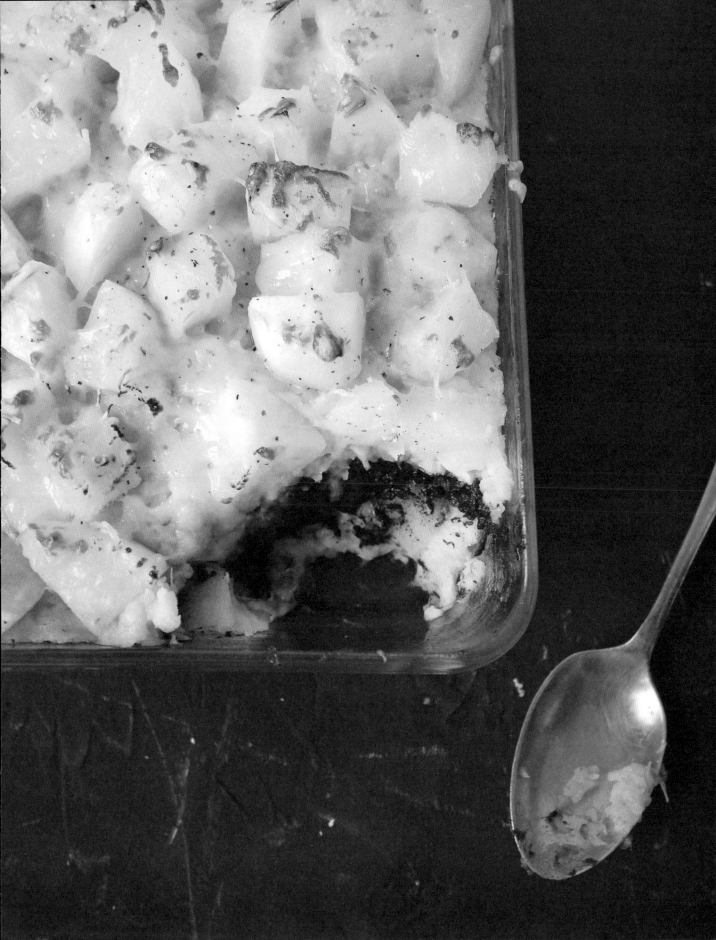

Crumbed haddock
WITH HERBS
cherry tomatoes + steamed zucchini

SERVES 2
PREPARATION TIME 30 MINUTES
COOKING TIME 15 MINUTES

Crumbed haddock with herbs

1 free-range egg
salt and freshly ground pepper
2 tablespoons breadcrumbs
2 tablespoons chopped flat-leaf
    (Italian) parsley
2 tablespoons chopped basil or
    coriander (cilantro)
1 tablespoon chopped chives or dill
4 haddock fillets, or substitute other
    firm, white-fleshed fish fillets
olive oil, for frying
fine sea salt, to finish

Cherry tomato salad with basil and steamed zucchini

2 zucchini (courgettes)
1 pinch of salt
1 dozen cherry tomatoes, halved
2 tablespoons olive oil
2 tablespoons balsamic vinegar

Lightly beat the egg in a shallow dish. Season with salt and pepper. Mix together the breadcrumbs and three-quarters of the herbs (keep some to scatter over the salad) in a second plate.

Dip both sides of the fish fillet in the egg, then in the breadcrumbs. Repeat the process with the remaining fish.

Heat a little olive oil and cook the fish fillets on a medium heat, about 4 minutes each side.

Make ribbons of zucchini with a peeler, keeping the skin. Place a glass of water in a saucepan with a pinch of salt and cook the zucchini, covered, over medium heat for 5 minutes. Drain.

On each plate, arrange a piece of crumbed fish, cherry tomatoes and zucchini ribbons. Dress with olive oil and balsamic vinegar and scatter with the remaining chopped herbs and fine sea salt.

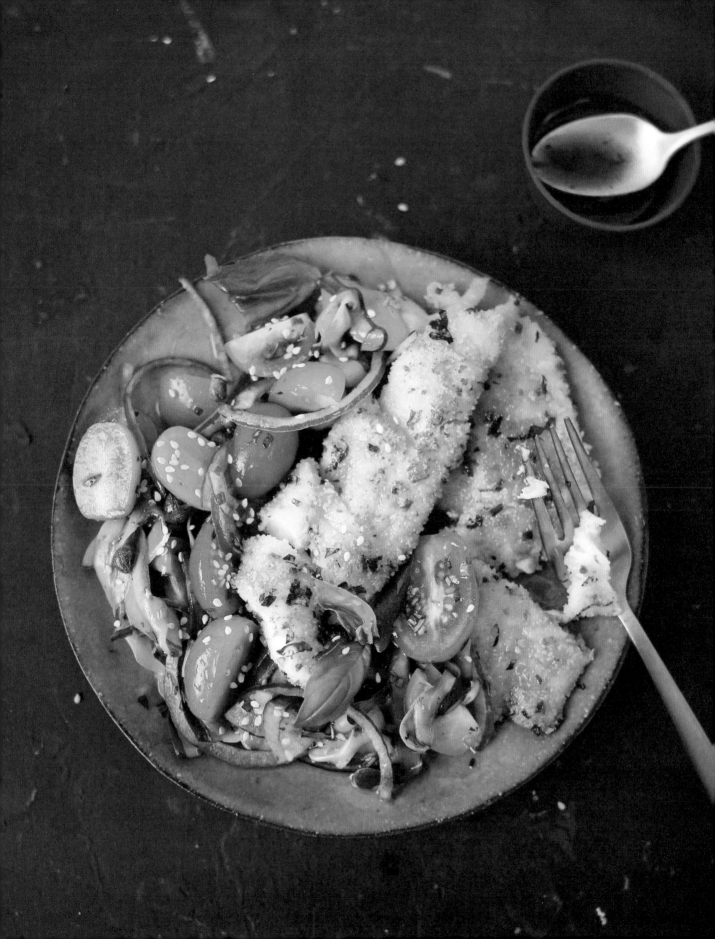

Tagliatelle
WITH VEGETABLES
zucchini + capsicum + cherry tomatoes

SERVES 2
PREPARATION TIME 15 MINUTES
COOKING TIME 20 MINUTES

1 zucchini (courgette), diced
1 capsicum (pepper), diced
1 dozen cherry tomatoes
2 garlic cloves, peeled and
   finely chopped
2 tablespoons olive oil
salt and pepper
1 teaspoon mixed dried herbs
   or dried oregano
300 g (10½ oz) fresh tagliatelle
   or wholemeal (whole-wheat) pasta
1 small bunch parsley, chopped
1 tablespoon sesame seeds

Preheat the oven to 210°C (425°F). Place the zucchini, capsicum and tomatoes in a large oven-proof dish or a baking tray lined with baking paper. Add the garlic, oil, salt, pepper and dried herbs and stir to coat the vegetables. Spread them out well so they are not on top of each other. Bake for about 20 minutes: the vegetables should be quite tender.

While the vegetables are cooking, cook the pasta in a saucepan of lightly salted boiling water until al dente. Drain the pasta and mix it with the vegetables in the dish. Scatter with parsley and sesame seeds before serving.

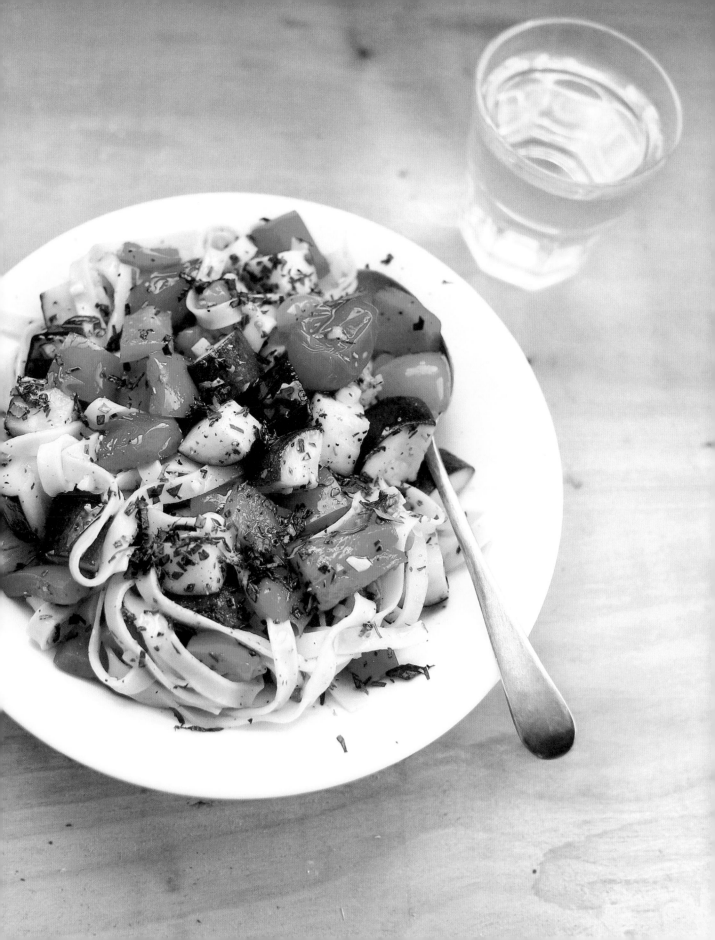

Grilled
SALMON
with green beans + lemon + tarragon + capers

SERVES 2
PREPARATION TIME 10 MINUTES
COOKING TIME 10–15 MINUTES

200 g (7 oz) thin green beans,
   trimmed, fresh or frozen
3 tablespoons olive oil for the
   marinade, plus extra, for frying
1 tablespoon balsamic vinegar
2 teaspoons baby capers
½ bunch tarragon, chopped
zest of 1 organic lemon
juice of 1 organic orange
15 g (½ oz) lightly salted butter
2 salmon fillets, about 100 g
   (3½ oz) each
sea salt, freshly ground pepper

Cook the beans in a saucepan of boiling salted water for 10–15 minutes, or until they are very tender. Drain and plunge into iced water. Drain again.

Combine the olive oil and a little balsamic vinegar in a bowl, then add the capers and tarragon. Pour this dressing over the green beans. Sprinkle with lemon zest and add the orange juice. Mix together and set aside in the refrigerator.

Pour a little olive oil in a hot frying pan, then add the butter. Place the salmon fillets in the frying pan, flesh side down. Season. Brown well, basting with the cooking fats. Turn the fillets over and baste again. When they are browned, place them on plates. Sprinkle with sea salt and freshly ground pepper. Serve with the green beans.

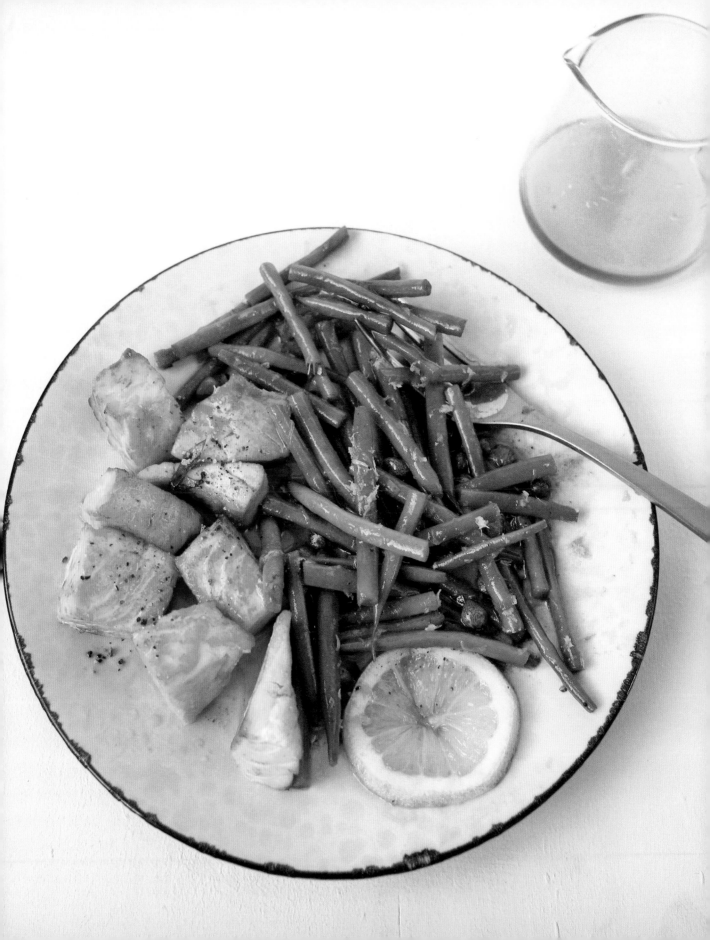

Vegetable
MINI PIZZAS
with artichoke + cherry tomatoes

SERVES 2
PREPARATION TIME 15 MINUTES
COOKING TIME 10 MINUTES

2–4 tablespoons olive oil
400 g (14 oz) tinned artichoke
  hearts, in brine or oil, drained
  and halved
70 g (2½ oz) cherry tomatoes, halved
fine sea salt
1 garlic clove, peeled and finely
  chopped, or 1 teaspoon
  garlic powder
1 roll pizza dough or 2 small balls of
  wholemeal (whole-wheat) pizza
  dough (see page 163)
4 tablespoons tomato passata
½ bunch flat-leaf (Italian) parsley
  (or basil), chopped

Preheat the oven to 250°C (500°F). Heat the oil in a frying pan over medium heat and sauté the artichoke hearts, cherry tomatoes and garlic.

On a floured surface, roll out the dough with a rolling pin. Make 2 rounds of dough. Spread 2 tablespoons of tomato passata on each round of dough. Divide the artichoke mixture between them and drizzle with a little olive oil.

Bake for about 10 minutes. When the pizzas come out of the oven, sprinkle with salt and parsley.

Recipe to aid digestion
A very light pizza, with lots of vegetables (artichokes in particular are high in fibre and help with digestion), a wholemeal (whole-wheat) base and no cheese!

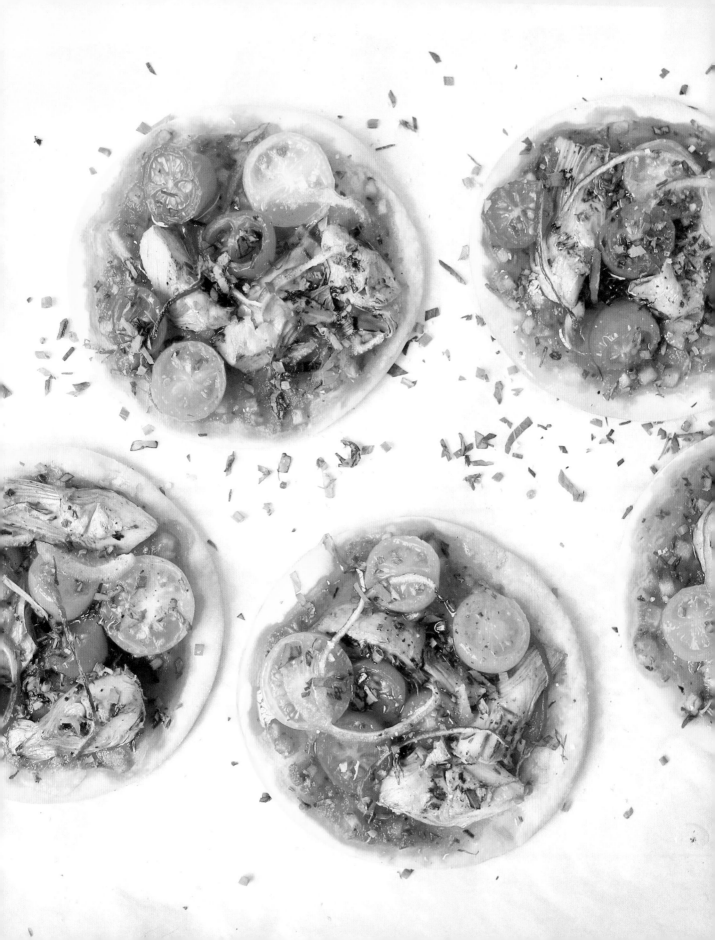

Handling
tricky situations

Cocktail hour

In the following pages you will learn how to control mojito frustration! You will also discover alternatives to (salty + fatty) potato crisps, canapés with caviar or slices of salami. Here's to a happy cocktail hour!

Afternoon snacks

It's hard not to dive into a packet of biscuits. To avoid giving in to this uncivilised habit, here are a few snack ideas that will satisfy your cravings for sweet things: light crêpes, mini yoghurt cakes, cookies with cereal and bananas.

Express meals

During pregnancy, you often have tired moments when you don't necessarily want to spend an hour in the kitchen cooking. And then sometimes you're suddenly hungry and waiting for something to simmer away is out of the question. At those times, the risk is to give in to ready-made meals that contain too much salt or sugar or, worse, a dinner of chocolate bars. And yet you can easily put together something tasty and healthy in 10 minutes. Here's proof.

Cocktail hour
PANTRY

A few ideas for nibbles to satisfy the salty-fatty-spicy cravings that typically go with "cocktail" hour.

Risks and temptations

ALCOHOL

No alcohol during pregnancy! This is one of the golden rules for a healthy baby.

SALT

You should also limit your salt (sodium) intake. Salt encourages water retention, which can lead to uncomfortable symptoms at the end of pregnancy (cramps, swollen feet, numb fingers). On the other hand, you need mineral salts like potassium and magnesium.

FAT

When you're avoiding cured meats, unpasteurised cheese or sushi and being cautious with raw foods, don't be tempted to dive into the potato chips.

Good alternatives

CRAVING SOMETHING CRUNCHY

- radishes + butter + salt + freshly ground pepper (or flavoured butter)
- halved mushrooms + olive oil + tarragon, garlic, lemon
- cherry tomatoes + caramel + poppy seeds

CRAVING PEANUTS

"Less fat — less salt" alternatives:
- edamame beans with 2 salts (sea salt flakes, flavoured or smoked salt)
- roasted almonds + honey + salt and pepper
- roasted pepitas (pumpkin seeds) + smoked salt

CRAVING SPICES

To replace the salty-spicy flavour of lots of shop-bought snacks:
- cooked broad beans + olive oil + paprika, garlic, cumin
- drained chickpeas + olive oil + Indian spice mix (or fenugreek)
- drained cannellini beans + olive oil + red pesto + pepper

CRAVING A WINE COOLER

- tomato juice + ground cumin
- grapefruit juice + 1 drop raspberry syrup

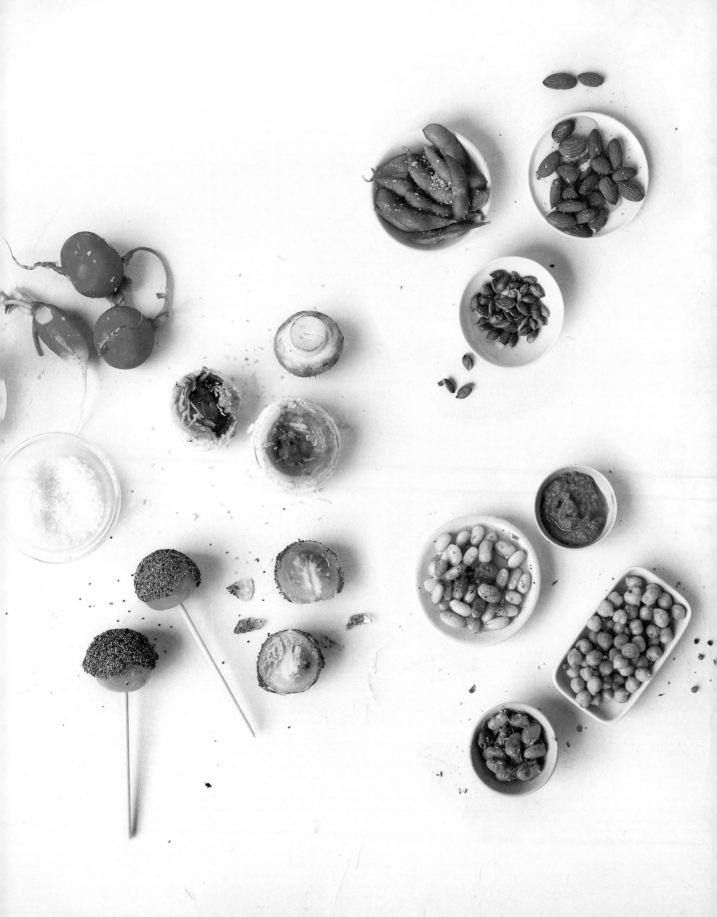

Virgin COCKTAILS

Being pregnant doesn't mean being cooped up at home.
You have a right to a social life! Especially since there
are alcohol-free versions of our favourite cocktails.

Virgin mojito

MAKES 2 GLASSES

4 tablespoons liquid sugar syrup
15–20 mint leaves, plus 2 tips, to garnish
2 organic limes, cubed
crushed ice or ice cubes, soda water

Pour the syrup into a tall, wide glass or cocktail shaker, add the mint leaves and the limes. Pound with a cocktail muddler or a large spoon. Add ice to two glasses and top up with soda water and the lime syrup. Mix well with a long spoon or a straw. Garnish with fresh mint tips.

Virgin spritz

MAKES 2 GLASSES

1 dash grenadine
500 ml (17 fl oz/2 cups) tonic water
1 organic orange, sliced into rounds
2 pieces organic grapefruit rind
a few ice cubes
2 green olives

Divide the grenadine and tonic water between two glasses and mix. Add some orange slices, grapefruit rind and ice cubes. Serve with a green olive on a toothpick, inserted into the grapefruit rind.

Virgin Long Island iced tea

MAKES 2 GLASSES

250 ml (9 fl oz/1 cup) iced tea (home-made
   or store-bought)
50 ml (1¾ fl oz) apple juice
50 ml (1¾ fl oz) organic lemon or lime juice
ice cubes, ginger beer or dry ginger ale

Mix together the iced tea, apple juice and lemon juice. Add some ice cubes and top up the glasses with ginger beer or ale.

Virgin cosmopolitan

MAKES 1 COCKTAIL PITCHER

125 ml (4 fl oz/½ cup) organic orange juice
500 ml (17 fl oz/2 cups) cranberry juice
3 tablespoons organic lime juice
1 dash of grenadine
250 ml (9 fl oz/1 cup) ginger beer or dry ginger ale
2 slices of organic lime, to garnish
crushed ice

Mix together the orange juice, cranberry juice, lime juice and grenadine in a pitcher. Add the ginger beer or ale and stir with a swizzle stick or straw. Serve in martini glasses with a slice of lime and crushed ice.

Virgin bloody mary

MAKES 1 GLASS

250 ml (9 fl oz/1 cup) tomato juice
1 teaspoon lemon juice
1 teaspoon Worcestershire sauce
1–2 drops Tabasco sauce
1 pinch of fine salt
1 pinch of pepper
1 pinch of celery salt
1 small celery stalk, to garnish

Pour the tomato juice, lemon juice, Worcestershire sauce and Tabasco into a large tall glass, and mix with a straw or a swizzle stick. Season with salt and pepper and celery salt. Place the celery stalk in the glass as a garnish.

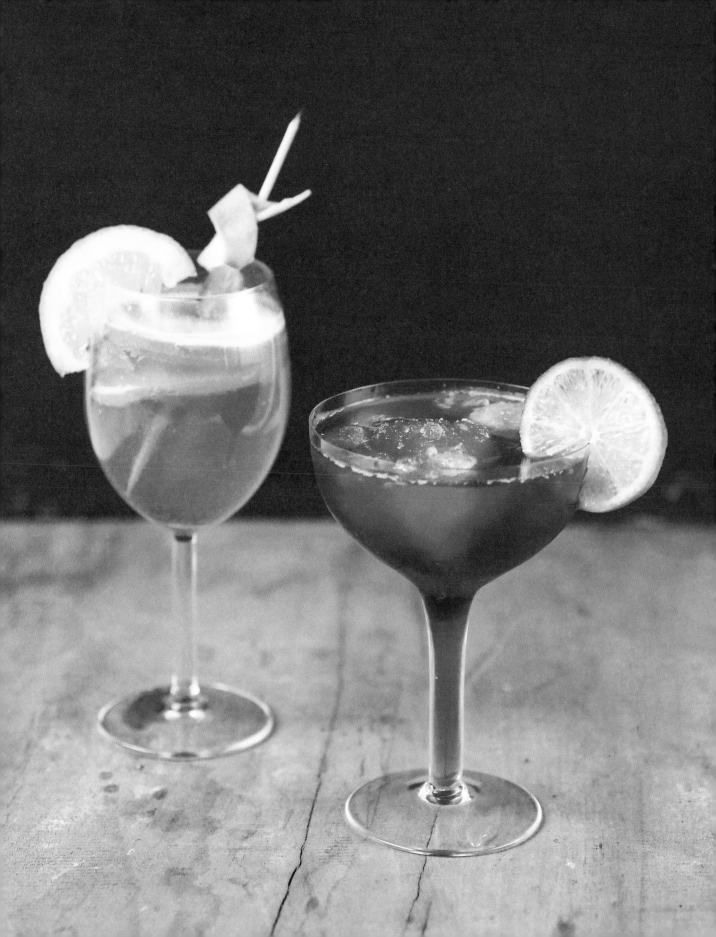

Healthy
DIPS

Tapenade with tahini

MAKES 1 BOWL
PREPARATION TIME 5 MINUTES
RESTING TIME 1 HOUR

150 g (5½ oz) black olives, pitted
2 tablespoons shelled walnuts
1 teaspoon tahini (sesame paste)
1 garlic clove, peeled
3–4 tablespoons olive oil
linseeds (flaxseeds)

In a food processor, purée the olives with the walnuts, tahini, garlic and olive oil. Season with pepper, sprinkle with linseeds. Rest the tapenade for 1 hour in the refrigerator before serving.

Guacamole with zucchini

MAKES 1 BOWL
PREPARATION TIME 10 MINUTES

2 ripe avocados, stones removed
1 small zucchini (courgette), cooked
    and sliced into rounds
1 tomato, diced
1 white onion, thinly sliced
1 drop Tabasco sauce
1 pinch of ground cumin
3 sprigs coriander (cilantro)
    and/or dill, chopped
juice of ½ organic lime or lemon
salt and freshly ground pepper

Cut open the avocados and remove the stone. In a large bowl, crush the avocado flesh and the zucchini with a fork, or purée in a food processor for a finer texture. Add the diced tomato, onion and Tabasco sauce and mix together well. Season with the cumin, lime juice, salt, pepper and add the herbs.

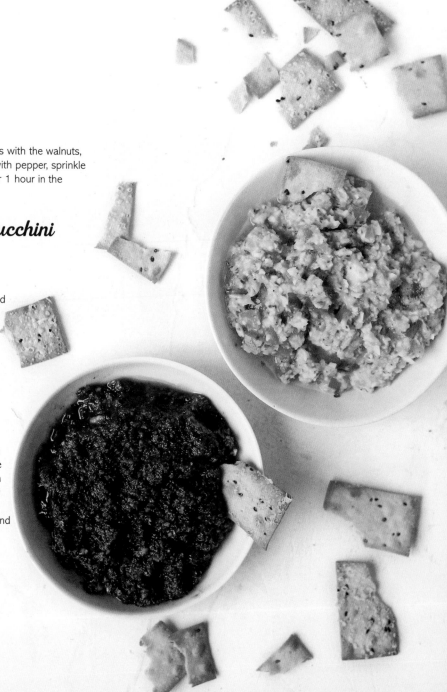

Omega-3 rillettes

MAKES 1 BOWL
PREPARATION TIME 15 MINUTES

110 g (3¾ oz) tinned sardines or mackerel, well drained
150 g (5½ oz) Philadelphia-style cream cheese
115 g (4 oz) mushrooms
juice of 1 organic lemon
1 tablespoon nutritional yeast flakes (from health
    food stores)
½ teaspoon salt, freshly ground pepper
¼ red onion, finely chopped (if using sardines)
    or the zest of 1 organic lime (if using mackerel)
1 tablespoon chopped chives
1 tablespoon chopped parsley

Process or mash all of the ingredients except the
herbs to a fluffy consistency. Add the herbs and
adjust the seasoning.

Serve with buckwheat blinis (see page 162).

CLASSIC VERSION: Use tinned tuna
in brine or springwater.

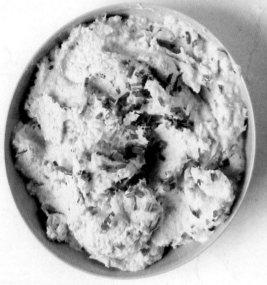
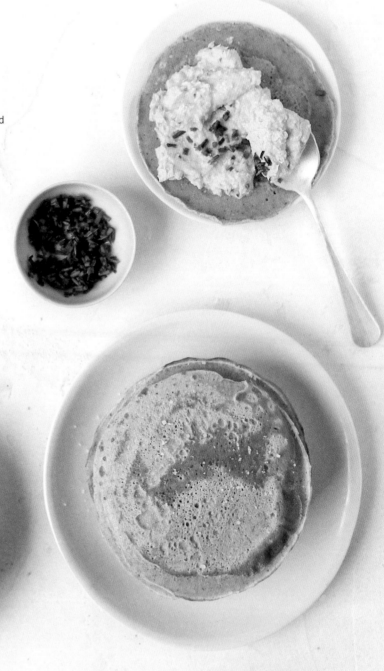

Mini
RICE PAPER ROLLS

MAKES 9 MINI RICE PAPER ROLLS
PREPARATION TIME 20 MINUTES
COOKING TIME 2–3 MINUTES

30 g (1 oz/1 sachet) rice vermicelli
    noodles
3 rice paper wrappers
2 carrots, peeled and grated
½ raw beetroot (beet), peeled
    and grated
9 mint leaves
1 avocado, thinly sliced
1 handful radish sprouts, well washed
sesame seeds, to sprinkle
sweet chilli sauce, to serve

Bring a saucepan of water to the boil. Immerse the rice vermicelli noodles in the boiling water for 2–3 minutes. Rinse under cold water and drain.

Place a shallow bowl of cold water on a work surface, with a clean, damp cloth beside it. Place 1 rice paper wrapper in the plate of cold water and let it soften for 1–2 minutes, until it becomes translucent and sticky, then lay it out on the damp cloth. Repeat with the remaining wrappers.

Divide the remaining ingredients between the wrappers, then close by folding the top and bottom edges towards the middle. Next, fold in the right edge. Roll up towards the left to make a roll. Cut each roll into three.

Serve with sweet chilli sauce and sprinkle with sesame seeds.

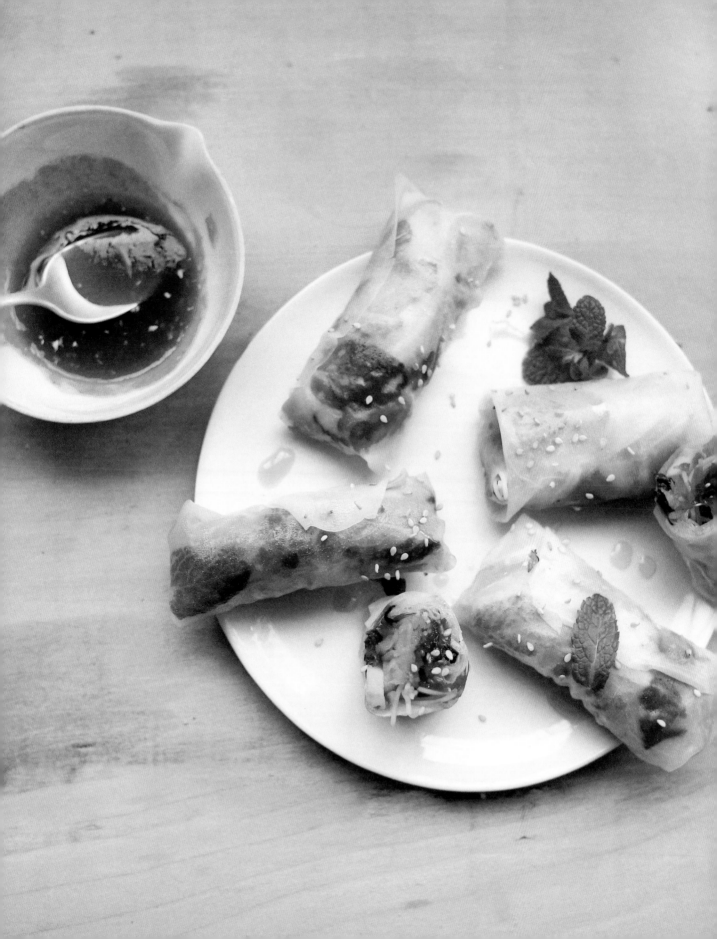

Mini pizzas
WITH LEMON

MAKES 6 MINI PIZZAS
PREPARATION TIME 15 MINUTES
COOKING TIME 10 MINUTES

1 roll pizza dough or 1 ball
   wholemeal (whole-wheat) pizza
   dough (see page 163)
3 organic lemons, sliced into very
   thin rounds.
dried oregano, as desired
3 teaspoons fennel seeds
50 ml (1¾ fl oz) olive oil
sea salt flakes and freshly ground
   pepper

Preheat the oven to 250°C (500°F). Roll out the pizza dough on a floured surface. Cut out circles 6–8 cm (2½–3¼ inches) in diameter until you run out of dough.

Place 1 slice of lemon on each circle. Sprinkle with dried oregano and fennel seeds. Drizzle with a little olive oil and sprinkle with salt flakes and pepper. Bake the pizzas for about 10 minutes and serve hot.

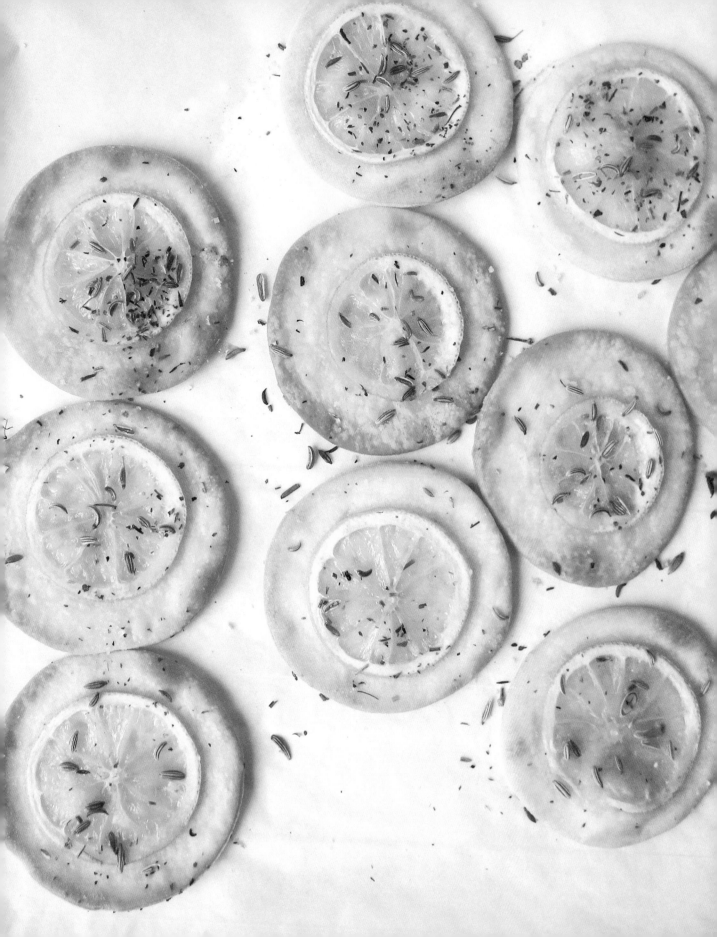

Bowl No.1
mixed salad + comté

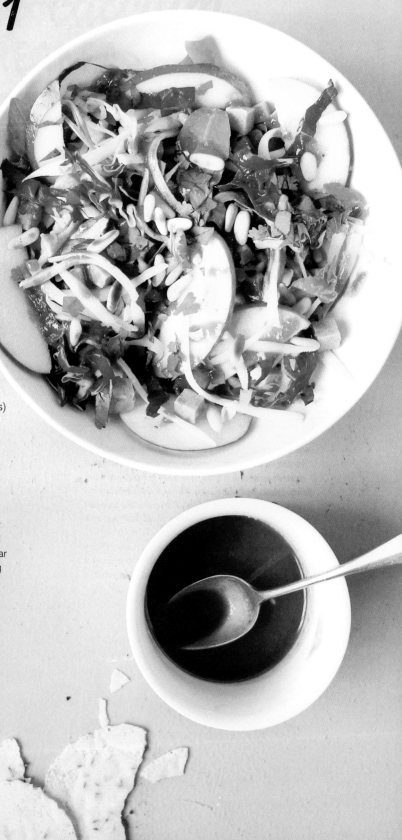

MAKES 1 LARGE BOWL
PREPARATION TIME 10 MINUTES

Salad

½ small radicchio lettuce, well washed
1 small handful rocket (arugula), well washed
½ pear (or ½ apple), thinly sliced
50 g (1¾ oz) aged comté or gruyère cheese,
   diced, shaved or cut into small sticks
50 g (1¾ oz) diced ham
1 tablespoon small chervil sprigs, to serve
1 tablespoon pine nuts (or shelled walnuts or pecans)
   to serve

Dressing

1 teaspoon balsamic vinegar
1 tablespoon olive oil
2 pinches of salt and freshly ground pepper
½ teaspoon tahini (sesame paste) (or sesame oil if
   you don't have tahini)

Cut the radicchio in half, then slice it thinly. In a salad
bowl, mix together the rocket, radicchio, slices of pear
(or apple), cheese and ham. Place all of the dressing
ingredients in a small jar and shake to combine.

To serve, pour the dressing over the salad and toss
together. Scatter with chervil and pine nuts.

Bowl No. 2

quinoa + grapefruit + avocado

MAKES 1 LARGE BOWL
PREPARATION TIME 10 MINUTES

Salad

60 g (2¼ oz) cooked quinoa
  (20 g [¾ oz] uncooked)
¼ fennel, sliced (choose a small bulb)
½ avocado, thinly sliced
1 small handful mâche lettuce, well washed
½ baby gem lettuce heart, well washed
  and thinly sliced
½ organic pink grapefruit, peeled, pith
  removed, cut into segments
3 cherry tomatoes, halved
1 small piece preserved lemon, very
  thinly sliced and chopped
1 handful mixed fresh herbs, such
  as parsley, chives, basil and/or
  coriander (cilantro), chopped

Dressing

1 teaspoon mustard
1 tablespoon cider vinegar
3 tablespoons olive oil
1 teaspoon maple syrup
salt and freshly ground pepper

Mix together the quinoa, fennel, avocado, lettuces, grapefruit and tomato
in a mixing bowl. Add the preserved lemon and the herbs. Place all of
the vinaigrette ingredients in a small jar and shake to combine.

To serve, pour the dressing over the salad and toss together.

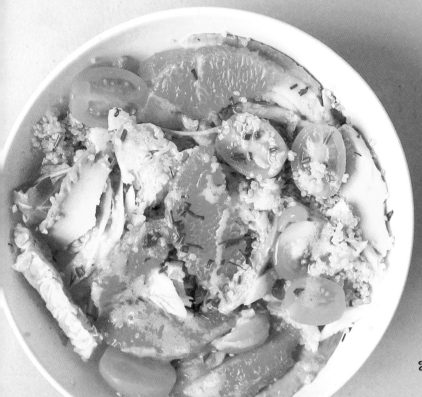

Express
STEAM BASKET
turkey + vegetables + tomato-coconut sauce

SERVES 2
PREPARATION TIME 5 MINUTES
COOKING TIME 20 MINUTES

2 small zucchini (courgettes), sliced
  into rounds
2 small carrots, cut into small sticks
1 small leek, white part only, cut in half
  and sliced
150 g (5½ oz) turkey escalope, sliced
  (or any white meat or fish fillet)
1 small handful coriander (cilantro)
  leaves, to serve

Steaming broth
1 litre (35 fl oz/4 cups) water
2 star anise
1 teaspoon turmeric or curry powder

Sauce
100 ml (3½ fl oz) coconut milk
1 teaspoon red curry paste
150 ml (5 fl oz) tomato passata
1 pinch of salt

To make the broth, place the water and spices in a saucepan that
will fit a lidded bamboo steamer basket on top. Bring to a simmer
over medium heat. Place the vegetables in the steamer basket,
cover and cook over the broth for 5 minutes. Add the turkey
and cook for a further 8 minutes (5–8 minutes if using fish).

Mix together the coconut milk with the curry paste in a small
saucepan and add the tomato passata and a pinch of salt.
Cook for 5 minutes on a low heat.

To serve, scatter the coriander leaves over the steamed turkey
and vegetables. Pour the sauce into a bowl and serve on the side.

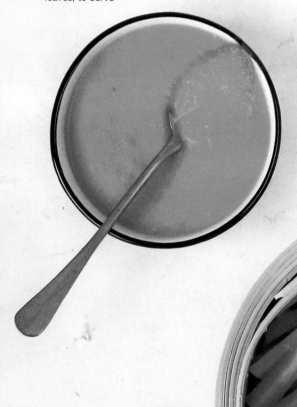

Express
SAUTÉ
spinach + chickpeas + eggs

SERVES 2
PREPARATION TIME 10 MINUTES
COOKING TIME 20 MINUTES

3 tablespoons olive oil
2 garlic cloves, peeled
1 teaspoon dried oregano, plus extra to garnish
½ teaspoon cumin
2 tomatoes, peeled and diced, or 150 ml (5 fl oz)
   tomato passata
300 g (10½ oz) tinned chickpeas, drained
200 ml (7 oz) chicken stock
salt and freshly ground pepper
120 g (4¼ oz) fresh spinach, or 80 g (2¾ oz)
   whole-leaf frozen spinach, thawed
2 free-range eggs

Heat the olive oil in a deep frying pan or wok over high heat, then sauté the garlic, dried oregano and cumin for a few minutes, until fragrant. Add the tomatoes and mix well. Add the chickpeas and chicken stock, season with salt and pepper and reduce the heat to a low simmer. Add the spinach, stir and cook for 5 minutes. Just before serving, remove the garlic. Break the eggs into the middle of the pan and scramble the yolks. Garnish with the extra oregano.

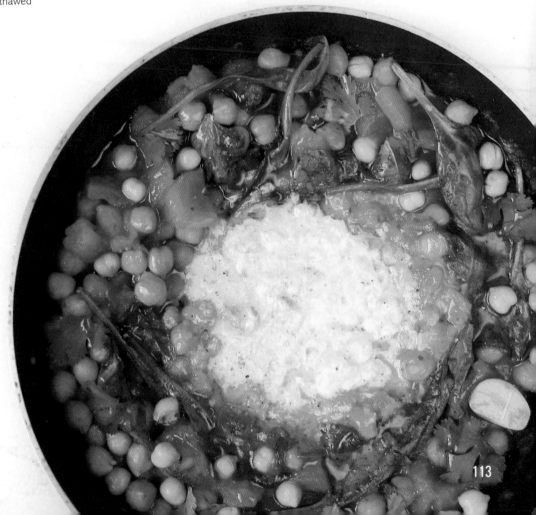

Express soup No. 1
WATERCRESS + POTATO

SERVES 2
PREPARATION TIME 10 MINUTES
COOKING TIME 20–25 MINUTES

1 bunch watercress
olive oil, for frying
1 garlic clove, peeled and crushed
1 potato, peeled and cut into large dice
600 ml (21 fl oz) water
1 teaspoon salt
1 teaspoon freshly ground pepper
1 organic vegetable stock cube
2 slices pain d'épice (French gingerbread)
  or any bread of choice, for toast

Wash the watercress in cold water and dry it in a salad
spinner. Cut off the base of the stems and keep the
tops. Heat the oil in a saucepan and lightly brown the
garlic and potato. Add the watercress, then the water,
salt, pepper and stock cube. Cook for 20–25 minutes,
over medium heat. Set aside a little of the cooking
liquid in a bowl. Blend the soup in a food processor,
adding the liquid to adjust if needed. Serve with toast.

Express gazpacho
TOMATO + ONION + CELERY

SERVES 2
PREPARATION TIME 10 MINUTES
COOKING TIME 25 MINUTES

5 large ripe tomatoes, diced
½ onion, peeled and sliced
1 celery stalk (or some fennel), diced
100 ml (3½ fl oz) water
1 slice wholemeal (whole-wheat) sandwich
  bread, torn into pieces, plus extra, for toast
50 ml (1¾ fl oz) olive oil, plus extra, to serve
1 tablespoon sherry vinegar
salt and freshly ground pepper
1 garlic clove, to serve

Blend the vegetables in a food processor on
maximum speed with the water, torn bread,
olive oil, vinegar, salt and pepper. Adjust the
consistency by adding more water, if necessary.

Rest the gazpacho in the refrigerator or serve at
room temperature, if preferred. To serve, pour into
serving bowls and top with a drizzle of olive oil.

Serve with wholemeal toast rubbed with garlic
and drizzled with extra olive oil.

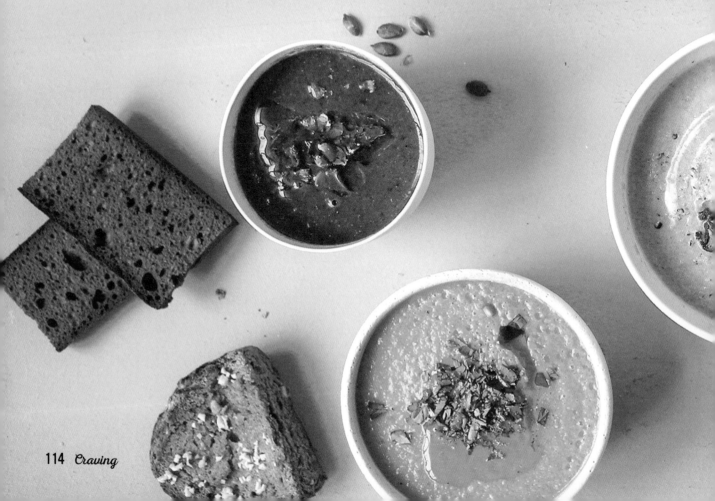

Express soup No. 2
MUSHROOM + CURRY

SERVES 2
PREPARATION TIME 10 MINUTES
COOKING TIME 20 MINUTES

500 g (1 lb 2 oz) mushrooms, well washed
1 tablespoon coconut oil (or olive oil)
1 large onion, peeled and thinly sliced
150 ml (5 fl oz) chicken stock
250 ml (9 fl oz/1 cup) pasteurised milk
100 ml (3½ fl oz) pouring cream (or coconut milk)
2 pinches of curry powder (or ground cumin or coriander)
salt and freshly ground pepper
chopped chervil and chives
2 multigrain rolls, to serve
spreadable goat's cheese, to serve

Roughly chop the mushrooms. Heat the oil in a saucepan and gently brown the onion with the mushrooms, stirring. Add the stock and simmer for 10 minutes. Add the milk, cream and curry powder. Season and simmer for a further 10 minutes. Blend the soup using a stick (hand-held) blender until as smooth as possible, then sprinkle with herbs.

Split the rolls, spread with goat's cheese and put under the grill for 10 minutes, then serve with the soup.

TIP: Cultivated, rather than wild, mushrooms are the most advisable to reduce the risk of toxoplasmosis.

Express soup No. 3
PUMPKIN + SWEET POTATO + COCONUT

SERVES 4
PREPARATION TIME 10 MINUTES
COOKING TIME 40 MINUTES

20 g (¾ oz) coconut oil or olive oil
½ red kuri or golden nugget pumpkin (squash), about 500 g (1 lb 2 oz), seeds removed and diced
300 g (10½ oz) sweet potato, peeled and diced
salt and freshly ground pepper
1 pinch each of cinnamon and nutmeg
2 sprigs thyme
2 teaspoons raw (demerara) sugar
200 ml (7 fl oz) coconut milk
Cheese Pastries: 4 tablespoons cream cheese + salt, pepper + 2 sheets brik pastry (or filo) cut in half + olive oil

Heat the coconut oil in a saucepan and sauté the vegetables. Add the salt, spices, thyme and sugar. Cover with water and simmer for 20 minutes.

Set aside a little of the cooking liquid in a bowl and remove the thyme. Blend the soup using a stick (hand-held) blender, adjusting the consistency if needed. Add the coconut milk and blend again.

To make the cheese pastries: season the cream cheese and place 1 tablespoon on each half-sheet of pastry. Fold pastry into a triangle. Heat olive oil in an ovenproof frying pan over medium-high heat and fry the triangles until lightly browned. Transfer to the oven and bake for 15 minutes at 200°C (400°F).

Serve the soup with cheese pastries on the side.

TIP: There's no need to peel the pumpkin if it is organic.

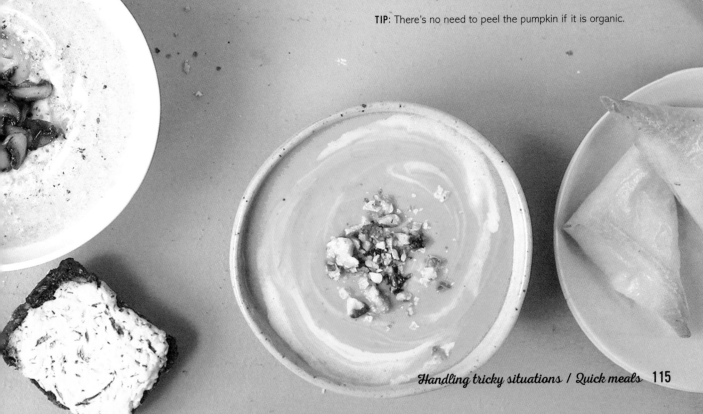

Macaroni
CHEESE
with eggplant

SERVES 2
PREPARATION TIME 10 MINUTES
COOKING TIME 30 MINUTES

olive oil, for frying
1 garlic clove, peeled and halved
1 eggplant (aubergine), diced
dried oregano or mixed herbs
250 ml (9 fl oz/1 cup) tomato passata
   (or tomato pasta sauce)
200 g (7 oz) macaroni or other
   short pasta
salt and freshly ground pepper
100 g (3½ oz) haloumi cheese,
   cut into large cubes (or a ball of
   mozzarella cheese)
parmesan cheese, grated

Preheat the oven to 180°C (350°F). Heat a little olive oil in a frying pan with the garlic. Sauté the eggplant for a few minutes, then remove the garlic, sprinkle with dried oregano and add the tomato passata.

Cook the macaroni in a large volume of salted water. Drain and add to the tomato sauce. Season to taste. Add the haloumi and pour everything into a small baking dish. Sprinkle with the parmesan and bake for 15–20 minutes, or until golden.

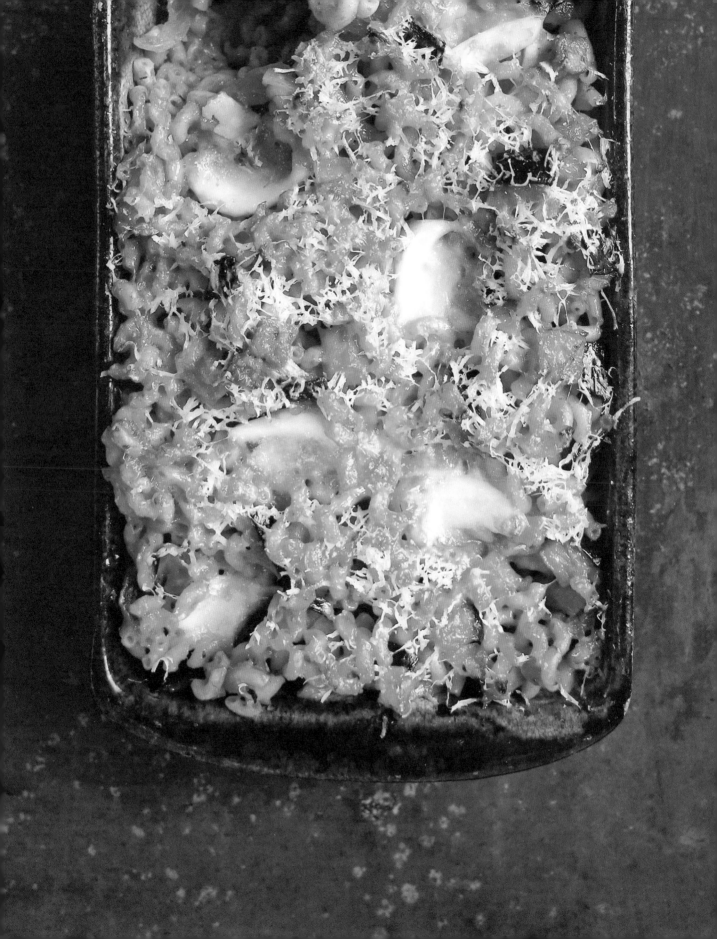

Japanese
RICE BOWL
Oyakodon

SERVES 2
PREPARATION TIME 10 MINUTES
COOKING TIME 15 MINUTES

2 teaspoons dashi (Japanese stock)
(or use fish sauce or fish stock)
1 leek, pale part only, thinly sliced
1 bulb spring onion (scallion)
(or yellow onion or sweet onion),
thinly sliced
150 g (5½ oz) chicken breast fillet,
sliced
2 teaspoons raw (demerara) sugar
2 tablespoons soy sauce
2 free-range eggs
200 g (7 oz) Japanese short-grain
rice, cooked
garlic chives, thinly sliced, to serve

Dilute the dashi in 100 ml (3½ fl oz) water in a deep frying pan. Heat gently and add the leek and onion. When they are soft and translucent, add the chicken. Add the sugar and soy sauce, mixing well, and sauté for 5 minutes.

Once the chicken is well cooked, lightly beat the eggs in a bowl and pour them over the chicken. Cover the frying pan with a lid, remove from the heat and leave to steam for 1 minute. Divide the rice between two bowls and arrange half of the chicken and vegetable omelette in each bowl. Sprinkle with garlic chives.

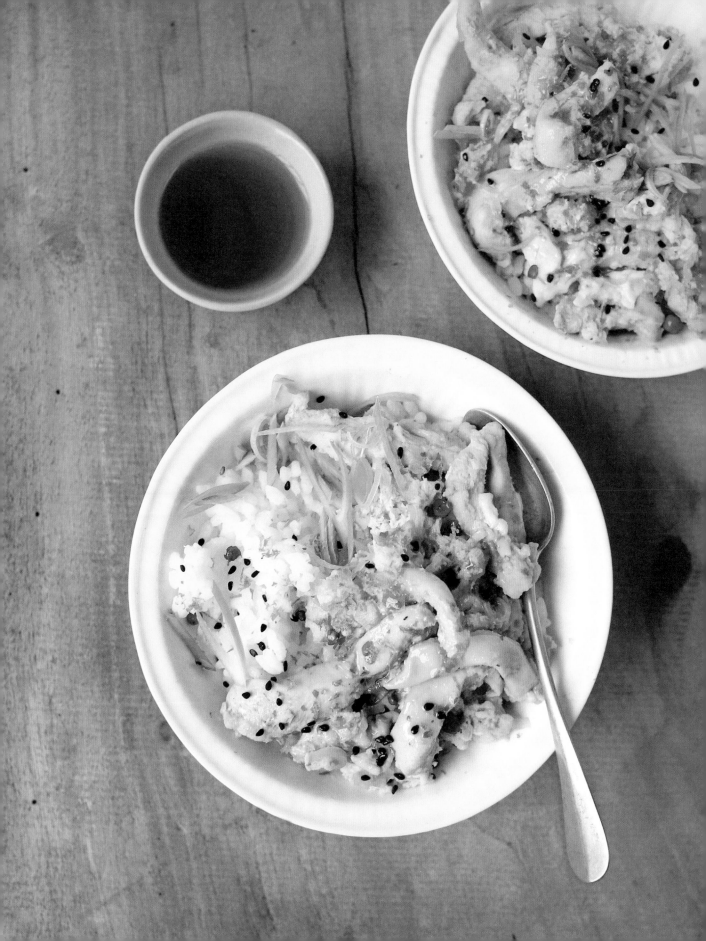

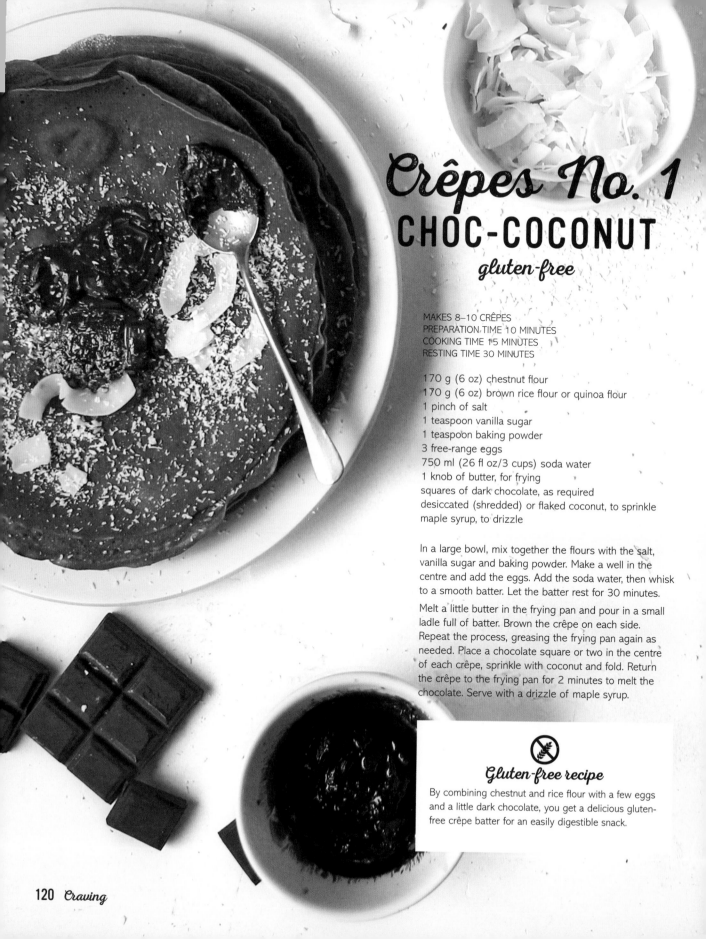

Crêpes No. 1
CHOC-COCONUT
gluten-free

MAKES 8–10 CRÊPES
PREPARATION TIME 10 MINUTES
COOKING TIME 15 MINUTES
RESTING TIME 30 MINUTES

170 g (6 oz) chestnut flour
170 g (6 oz) brown rice flour or quinoa flour
1 pinch of salt
1 teaspoon vanilla sugar
1 teaspoon baking powder
3 free-range eggs
750 ml (26 fl oz/3 cups) soda water
1 knob of butter, for frying
squares of dark chocolate, as required
desiccated (shredded) or flaked coconut, to sprinkle
maple syrup, to drizzle

In a large bowl, mix together the flours with the salt, vanilla sugar and baking powder. Make a well in the centre and add the eggs. Add the soda water, then whisk to a smooth batter. Let the batter rest for 30 minutes.

Melt a little butter in the frying pan and pour in a small ladle full of batter. Brown the crêpe on each side. Repeat the process, greasing the frying pan again as needed. Place a chocolate square or two in the centre of each crêpe, sprinkle with coconut and fold. Return the crêpe to the frying pan for 2 minutes to melt the chocolate. Serve with a drizzle of maple syrup.

Gluten-free recipe

By combining chestnut and rice flour with a few eggs and a little dark chocolate, you get a delicious gluten-free crêpe batter for an easily digestible snack.

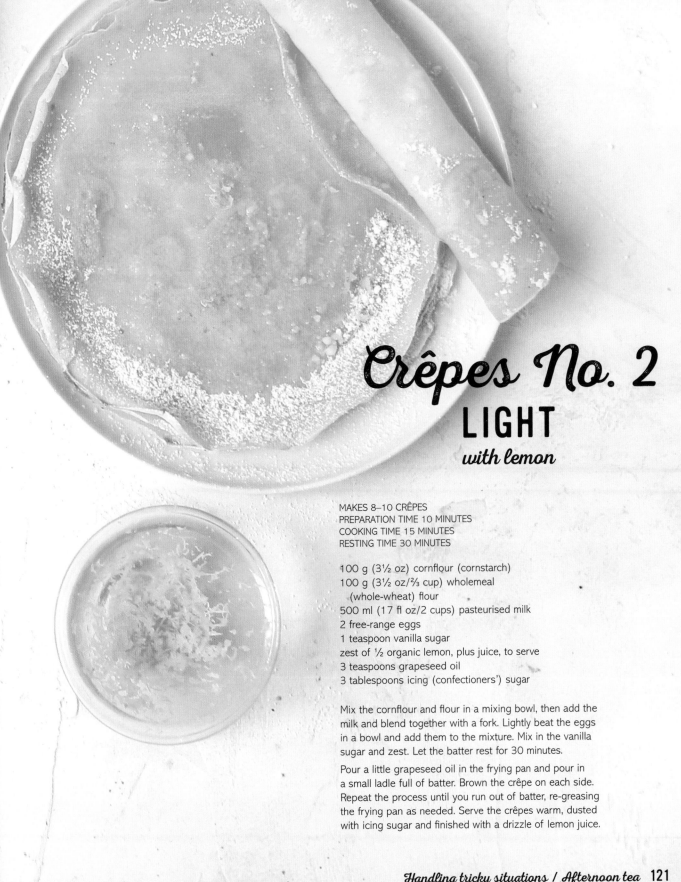

Crêpes No. 2
LIGHT
with lemon

MAKES 8–10 CRÊPES
PREPARATION TIME 10 MINUTES
COOKING TIME 15 MINUTES
RESTING TIME 30 MINUTES

100 g (3½ oz) cornflour (cornstarch)
100 g (3½ oz/⅔ cup) wholemeal
  (whole-wheat) flour
500 ml (17 fl oz/2 cups) pasteurised milk
2 free-range eggs
1 teaspoon vanilla sugar
zest of ½ organic lemon, plus juice, to serve
3 teaspoons grapeseed oil
3 tablespoons icing (confectioners') sugar

Mix the cornflour and flour in a mixing bowl, then add the milk and blend together with a fork. Lightly beat the eggs in a bowl and add them to the mixture. Mix in the vanilla sugar and zest. Let the batter rest for 30 minutes.

Pour a little grapeseed oil in the frying pan and pour in a small ladle full of batter. Brown the crêpe on each side. Repeat the process until you run out of batter, re-greasing the frying pan as needed. Serve the crêpes warm, dusted with icing sugar and finished with a drizzle of lemon juice.

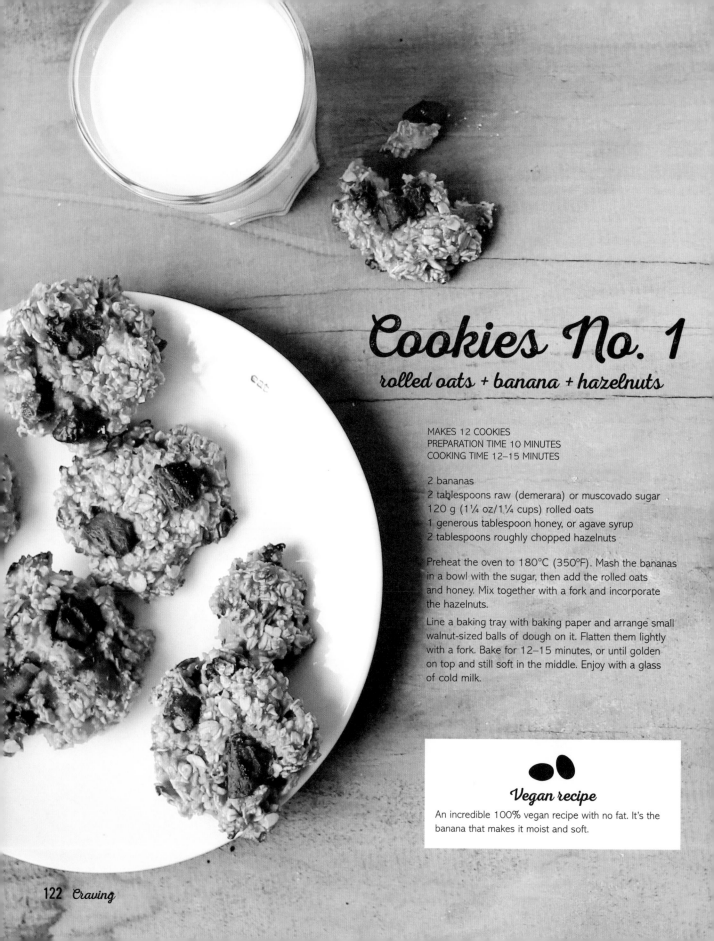

Cookies No. 1
rolled oats + banana + hazelnuts

MAKES 12 COOKIES
PREPARATION TIME 10 MINUTES
COOKING TIME 12–15 MINUTES

2 bananas
2 tablespoons raw (demerara) or muscovado sugar
120 g (1¼ oz/1¼ cups) rolled oats
1 generous tablespoon honey, or agave syrup
2 tablespoons roughly chopped hazelnuts

Preheat the oven to 180°C (350°F). Mash the bananas in a bowl with the sugar, then add the rolled oats and honey. Mix together with a fork and incorporate the hazelnuts.

Line a baking tray with baking paper and arrange small walnut-sized balls of dough on it. Flatten them lightly with a fork. Bake for 12–15 minutes, or until golden on top and still soft in the middle. Enjoy with a glass of cold milk.

Vegan recipe

An incredible 100% vegan recipe with no fat. It's the banana that makes it moist and soft.

Cookies No. 2
cranberries + white chocolate

MAKES 10 COOKIES
PREPARATION TIME 10 MINUTES
COOKING TIME 15 MINUTES

120 g (4¼ oz) butter, softened
180 g (6½ oz) sugar
1 free-range egg
1 level teaspoon bicarbonate of soda
   (baking soda)
1 tablespoon liquid vanilla extract
½ teaspoon salt
200 g (7 oz) wholemeal (whole-wheat)
   flour (or a combination of quinoa and
   rice flour)
50 g (1¾ oz) dried cranberries,
   finely chopped
100 g (3½ oz) white chocolate chips
   (optional)

Preheat the oven to 150°C (300°F). Mix the
butter with the sugar using a spatula. Add
the egg, bicarb, vanilla extract and salt. Mix
together well and gradually incorporate the
flour. Mix in the cranberries and chocolate
chips by hand or with the spatula.

Line a baking tray with baking paper.
Arrange small walnut-sized balls of
dough on the tray, spacing them well.
Bake for 15 minutes. Serve warm.

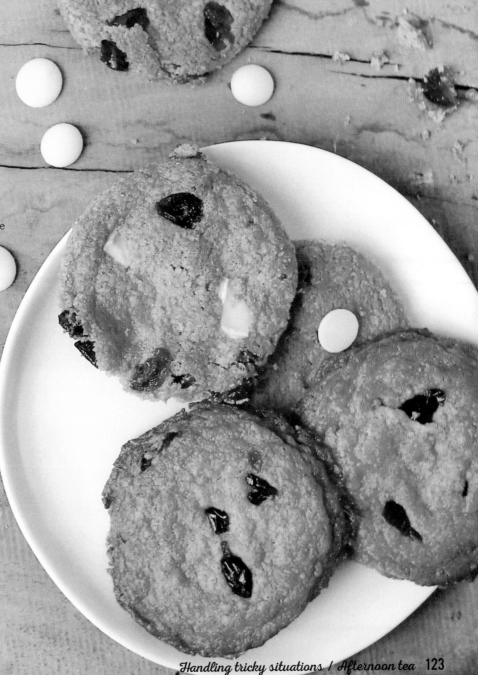

Cupcake No. 1

blueberry muffin

MAKES 12 MUFFINS
PREPARATION TIME 15 MINUTES
COOKING TIME 25 MINUTES

butter, for greasing
100 ml (3½ fl oz) canola or grapeseed oil
3 free-range eggs
100 ml (3½ fl oz) milk
250 g (9 oz) raw (demerara) or light brown sugar
zest of ½ organic lemon
350 g (12 oz/2⅓ cups) plain (all-purpose) flour
1 teaspoon baking powder
½ teaspoon bicarbonate of soda (baking soda)
½ teaspoon salt
300 g (10½ oz) fresh or frozen blueberries, thawed
2 teaspoons poppy seeds
icing (confectioners') sugar, for dusting

Preheat the oven to 180°C (350°F) and lightly grease a
12-hole muffin tin. In a mixing bowl, beat the oil with the
eggs and milk. Add the sugar and beat until the batter is
nice and creamy. Mix in the zest, flour, baking powder,
bicarb and salt. Add the blueberries and stir them in gently
so you don't crush them.

Fill the muffin moulds to three-quarters full, sprinkle with
poppy seeds and bake for 25 minutes. Let them cool on
a rack, then dust with icing sugar.

VARIATION: Replace the lemon zest with 2 stems
of lemongrass: crush them to a pulp using a
mortar and pestle and mix in to the batter.

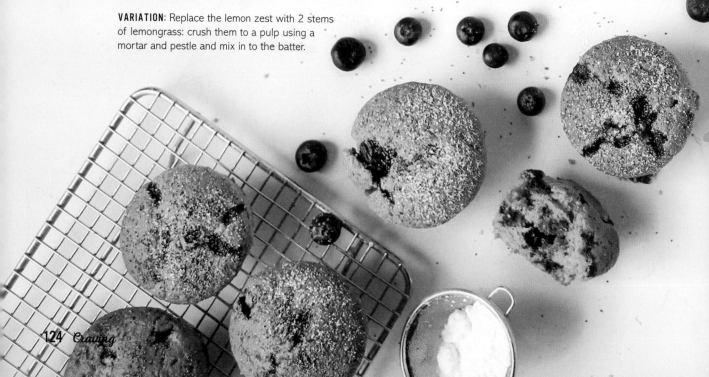

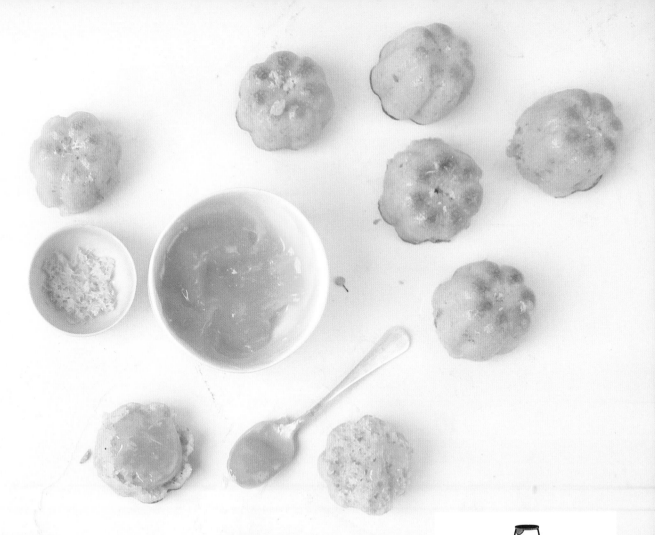

Cupcake No. 2
yoghurt + lemon curd cake

Special calcium recipe

Moist, lemony, calcium-rich. An ideal second trimester snack.

MAKES 6 MINI-CAKES
PREPARATION TIME 15 MINUTES
COOKING TIME 10–15 MINUTES

125 g (4½ oz/1 small tub) plain
   yoghurt
200 g (9 oz/1 cup) raw (demerara)
   sugar
1 pinch of salt
10 g (¼ oz/2 teaspoons) baking
   powder
150 g (5½ oz/1 cup) plain flour
50 g (1¾ oz/ 1 cup) ground almonds
3 eggs
zest of 1 organic lemon
30 g (1 oz) butter, melted, plus extra,
   for greasing
100 g (3½ oz) lemon curd

Preheat the oven to 180°C (350°F). In a mixing bowl, mix together the yoghurt with the sugar, salt, baking powder and sifted flour until well combined. Mix in the ground almonds, eggs, zest and melted butter — make sure the butter isn't too hot.

Pour the batter into small buttered moulds and bake for 10–15 minutes, depending on the mould used: they should be just brown.

Let the cakes cool, then cut them in two horizontally and spread lemon curd on top.

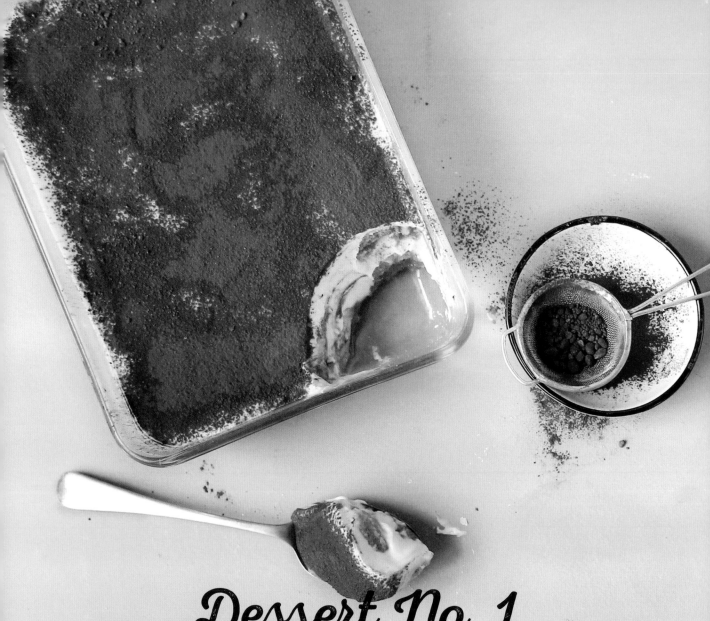

Dessert No. 1
light tiramisu (no eggs!)

MAKES 1 SMALL DISH
PREPARATION TIME 10 MINUTES
RESTING TIME 30 MINUTES–1 HOUR

150 ml (5 fl oz) water
2 tablespoons sugar
1 teaspoon instant coffee
400 g (14 oz) fromage blanc (see Tip)
160 g (5¾ oz/⅔ cup) mascarpone cheese
70 g (2½ oz) icing (confectioners') sugar
1 teaspoon vanilla sugar
15 ladyfinger biscuits
unsweetened cocoa powder

Mix together the water, sugar and coffee extract in a shallow bowl. In another bowl, beat together the fromage blanc and mascarpone, icing sugar and vanilla sugar. Dip 2–3 ladyfinger biscuits in the coffee mixture, then lay them in the bottom of a small serving dish. Top with a layer of mascarpone mixture, then 2–3 dipped ladyfingers, and another layer of the mixture. Dust with cocoa powder. Refrigerate the tiramisu for 30 minutes to 1 hour before serving.

TIP: If fromage blanc is unavailable, substitute labneh (hung yoghurt cheese), quark or thick Greek yoghurt.

Dessert No. 2

hazelnut fondant cakes

MAKES 4 CAKES
PREPARATION TIME 10 MINUTES
COOKING TIME 15 MINUTES

180 g (6½ oz) butter, plus extra,
  for greasing
160 g (5¾ oz/1½ cups) ground
  hazelnuts
45 g (1¾ oz/⅓ cup) wholemeal
  (whole-wheat) flour
1 generous tablespoon cocoa
  powder
4 free-range eggs
120 g (4¼ oz/1 cup) icing
  (confectioners') sugar
3 tablespoons unsweetened
  evaporated milk
4 squares of hazelnut or praline
  chocolate
4 teaspoons hazelnut butter
a few chopped hazelnuts
vanilla ice cream, to serve

Preheat the oven to 180°C (350°F). Melt the butter in a saucepan over a low heat, or in a bowl in a microwave oven, then let it cool a little. Combine the ground hazelnuts with the flour and cocoa powder in a mixing bowl. Stir in the melted butter. Mix in the eggs, one at a time, then the icing sugar and evaporated milk.

Butter four small moulds and fill them with the batter. Place 1 square of chocolate and 1 teaspoon of hazelnut butter in the middle of each. Bake for 15 minutes. Let them cool a little and sprinkle with chopped hazelnuts. Serve warm, with a scoop of vanilla ice cream.

I'm craving...

Pickles, tagines, burgers, taramasalata, chocolate… Something fatty, sugary or spicy. Strange and powerful cravings can start from the second trimester. Don't ever ignore a craving because it can turn into a frustration and then you risk overcompensating. It's important to give in to temptation as long as it is safe to do so. And this book is here to help you do just that.

On the following pages are some simple recipes that will allow you to satisfy those cravings, without going off the rails, overdoing it or getting frustrated. I've included alternatives to some foods that are currently off-limits, as well as reduced butter/reduced sugar versions of recipes, and healthy options for some popular dishes. Read on for the answers to your food prayers.

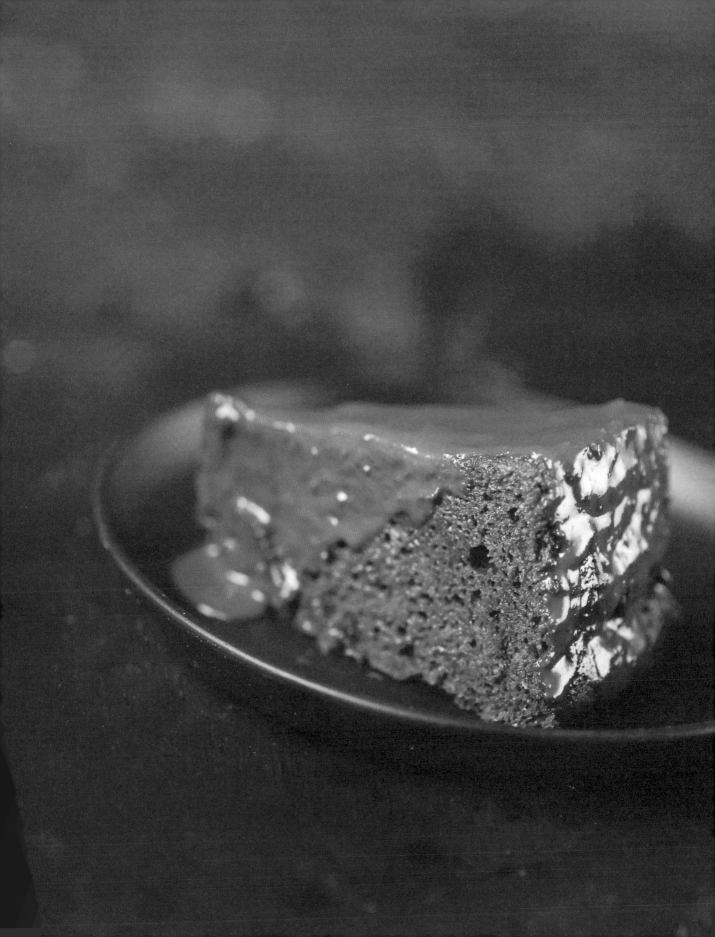

Gluten-free brownies
CHOCOLATE + SWEET POTATO

MAKES 1 TRAY OF BROWNIES
PREPARATION TIME 15 MINUTES
COOKING TIME 25 MINUTES

100 g (3½ oz) margarine (or soft butter or coconut oil),
   plus extra, for greasing
140 g (5 oz) milk (or dark) chocolate
140 g (5 oz) sweet potato purée
125 g (4½ oz) coconut sugar or muscovado sugar
2 free-range eggs
2 teaspoons liquid vanilla extract
½ teaspoon salt
100 g (3½ oz) white rice flour
2 tablespoons cornflour (cornstarch)
1 handful roughly chopped pecans

Preheat the oven to 180°C (350°F). Lightly grease a
brownie tray with a little margarine. Melt the margarine
and the chocolate in a small saucepan on a low heat.
Allow to cool slightly. In a large bowl, beat the sweet
potato purée with the coconut sugar, eggs, vanilla and
salt. Add the melted chocolate, in a thin stream, while
mixing with a spatula. Add the rice flour and cornflour.
Mix together well. Stir in the nuts. Pour into the tray and
cook for 20–25 minutes. Allow to cool before cutting.

Chocolate mousse
RAW EGG-FREE

MAKES 2 MOUSSES
PREPARATION TIME 15 MINUTES RESTING TIME 4 HOURS

150 g (5½ oz) good-quality dark cooking chocolate
   (or half dark and half milk)
100 ml (3½ fl oz) pasteurised milk
100 ml (3½ fl oz) thickened (whipping) cream
2 tablespoons honey
2 squares milk chocolate, chopped, to serve

Place the chocolate, broken into squares, in a mixing bowl.
In a small saucepan, bring the milk to the boil and pour
it over the squares of chocolate. After a few seconds,
beat together with a whisk until shiny. Allow to cool.

For the whipped cream: place a glass mixing bowl and
the beater attachments of an electric beater in the
freezer 30 minutes in advance. Pour the cream into the
mixing bowl and beat. It should double in volume.

Gently combine the chocolate and whipped cream with
a spatula. Pour into small individual pots, cover with plastic
wrap and let them set in the refrigerator for 2 hours.
At serving time, sprinkle with the chopped chocolate.

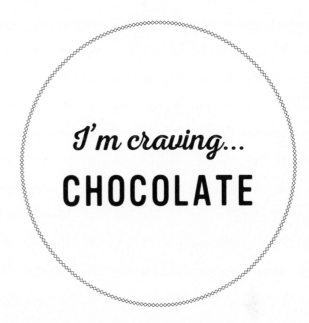

I'm craving...
CHOCOLATE

Chocolate fondant cake
WITH LIGHT ICING

MAKES A 20 CM (8 INCH)
PREPARATION TIME 15 MINUTES
COOKING TIME 20 MINUTES
RESTING TIME 30 MINUTES

250 g (9 fl oz) good-quality dark cooking chocolate
4 free-range eggs, separated
40 g (1½ oz) rapadura sugar (or light brown sugar)
15 g (½ oz) cornflour (cornstarch)
100 g (3½ oz) fromage blanc, or substitute quark or
   labneh (hung yoghurt cheese)
1 teaspoon baking powder
1 pinch of salt

Icing
150 ml (5½ fl oz) almond milk
100 g (3½ oz) good quality dark or milk cooking chocolate
2 tablespoons agave or maple syrup

Preheat the oven to 180°C (350°F). Melt the chocolate in
a double boiler. In a mixing bowl, beat the egg yolks with the
sugar. Once the mixture is pale and light, add the cornflour,
fromage blanc, baking powder, salt and melted chocolate.
Mix together to a smooth batter. Beat the egg whites to soft
peaks. Gently fold them into the batter. Butter a spring-form
cake tin, pour in the batter and bake for 20 minutes. Allow to
cool a little before unmoulding.

For the icing: heat the milk, removing from the heat just before
it comes to the boil. Add the chocolate, in pieces, and mix until
smooth. Mix in the syrup and cool for 10 minutes to thicken.
Pour the icing over the cake and refrigerate for 30 minutes.

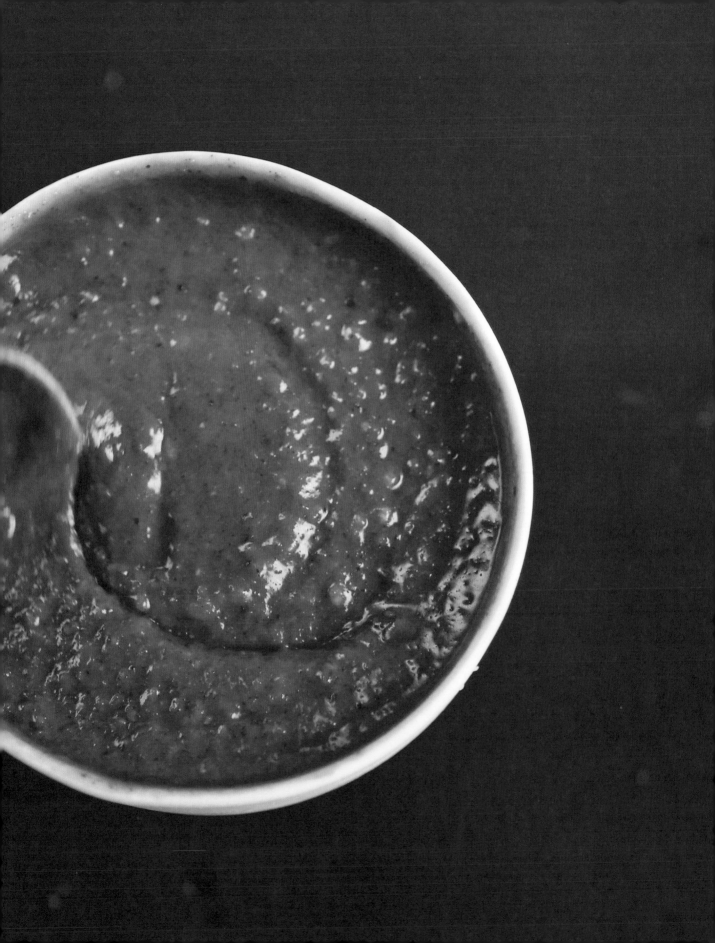

Choc-hazelnut
SPREAD

MAKES 1 JAR SPREAD
PREPARATION TIME 10 MINUTES

160 g (5¾ oz) good-quality milk chocolate, in pieces
50 ml (1¾ fl oz) almond milk (or semi-skimmed
  pasteurised milk)
20 g (¾ oz) agave syrup or honey (optional)
90 g (3¼ oz) ground hazelnuts (or ground almonds)
1 generous tablespoon of organic hazelnut butter

Heat the chocolate in a double-boiler with the milk
and stir with a fork. Add the agave syrup (if using),
then the ground hazelnuts and hazelnut butter.

Pour into a sterilised jam jar and serve immediately or let it
cool before refrigerating. Keeps, refrigerated, for one week.

TIP: For a less sweet version, mix together 1 teaspoon of
unsweetened cocoa powder with 1 teaspoon of honey,
1 teaspoon of ground hazelnuts and 1 teaspoon of
pasteurised milk in a bowl.

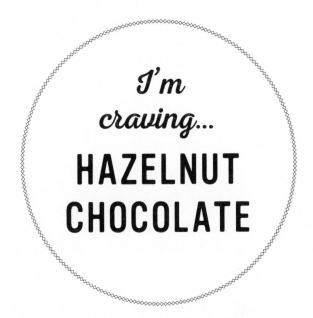

I'm craving...
HAZELNUT CHOCOLATE

Wafer roll biscuits
WITH CHOC-HAZELNUT SPREAD

MAKES 6 ROLLS
PREPARATION TIME 15 MINUTES
COOKING TIME 20 MINUTES

1 packet of filo pastry
100 g (3½ oz) home-made choc-hazelnut spread
  (see above), or store-bought equivalent (or 60 g [2¼ oz]
  melted chocolate and 40 g [1½ oz] hazelnut butter)
1 small handful flaked almonds
1 free-range egg yolk

Preheat the oven to 180°C (350°F). Lay 10 sheets of filo
pastry on a work surface. Cut out a large 30 cm x 30 cm
(12 inch x 12 inch) square, then 8 cm x 30 cm (3¼ inch
x 12 inch) strips. Cover the strips with the spread and roll
them up into cigars. Pinch the ends with your fingertips.

Place the cigars on a baking tray lined with baking paper.
Brush with beaten egg and sprinkle with flaked almonds.
Bake for 20 minutes.

These biscuits are delicious hot, warm or cold, dipped in
more choc-hazelnut spread.

Pure energy truffles
HONEY + HAZELNUTS + COCONUT

MAKES 15 TRUFFLES
PREPARATION TIME 15 MINUTES
RESTING TIME 30 MINUTES

100 g (3½ oz) rolled oats
2 tablespoons home-made choc-hazelnut spread (see
  above) or store-bought equivalent
2 tablespoons desiccated (shredded) coconut
2 teaspoons honey
3 tablespoons of unblanched shelled hazelnuts, toasted,
  or hazelnut butter
2 tablespoons liquid vanilla extract
1 pinch of salt
3 tablespoons agave syrup

Grind all the ingredients together in a food processor.
Rest the processed mixture in the refrigerator for 30 minutes
to firm it. Shape into small 2 cm (¾ inch) balls like truffles.
Leave to rest in the refrigerator until serving time.

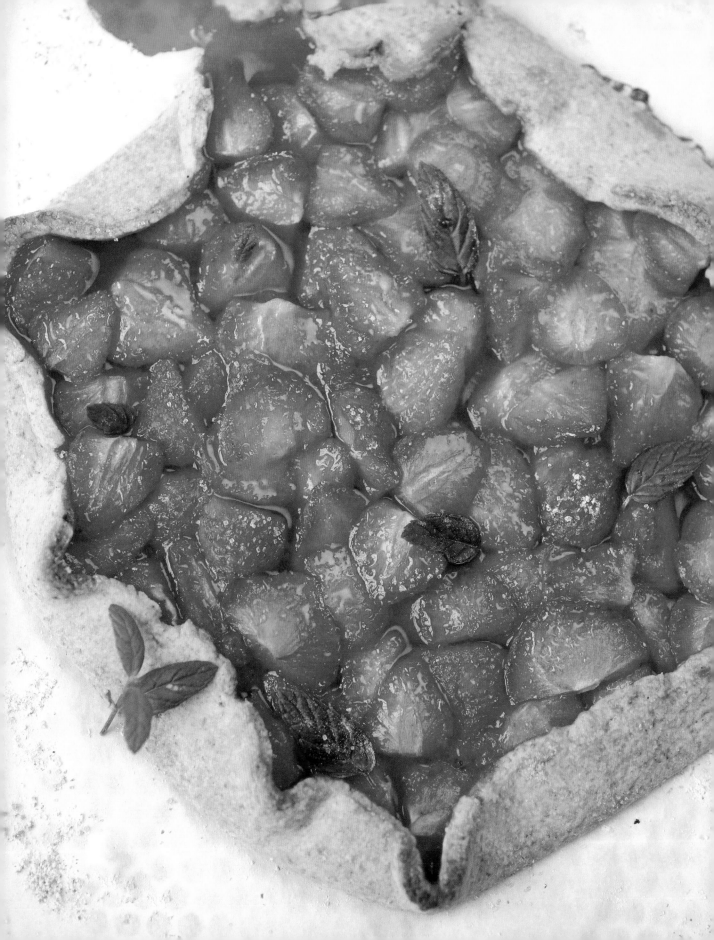

Rustic tartlets
STRAWBERRIES + FROMAGE BLANC

MAKES 4 TARTLETS
PREPARATION TIME 20 MINUTES
COOKING TIME 25 TO 30 MINUTES   RESTING TIME 15 MINUTES

Pastry dough
200 g (7 oz/1⅓ cups) wholemeal (whole-wheat) flour
  (or half plain [all-purpose] flour, half wholemeal flour)
60 g (2¼ oz) raw (demerara) sugar
1 pinch of salt
1 free-range egg yolk
60 g (2¼ oz) unsalted butter, softened
60 g (2¼ oz) fromage blanc, or quark or labneh
  (hung yoghurt cheese)

Filling
500 g (1 lb 2 oz) strawberries, thinly sliced
3 tablespoons flour
3 tablespoons light brown sugar
icing (confectioners') sugar, to sprinkle

Preheat the oven to 180°C (350°F). Combine the strawberries with the flour and sugar in a mixing bowl.

For the pastry, mix together the flour, sugar and salt in a bowl. Add the butter and rub in with your fingertips until the dough resembles crumbs. Mix in the egg yolk and 2 tablespoons of cold water: the dough should form a smooth ball. Roll onto a floured surface and cut out four circles, 14 cm (5½ inches) in diameter. Place them in the refrigerator for 15 minutes.

Place the circles of pastry on a baking tray lined with baking paper. Spoon 2–3 tablespoons of strawberry filling in the centres, leaving a 2 cm (¾ inch) border. Fold in the edges to make a crust. Bake for 25–30 minutes: the pastry should be golden. Let the tartlets cool before dusting with icing sugar.

Avocado-strawberry open sandwiches
CUCUMBER + CORIANDER

MAKES 2 OPEN SANDWICHES   PREPARATION TIME 10 MINUTES

2 tablespoons olive oil
2 large slices of dark rye bread
1 avocado, thinly sliced
¼ cucumber, sliced into rounds
salt and freshly ground pepper
4 strawberries, thinly sliced
2 tablespoons agave or maple syrup
2 coriander (cilantro) leaves

Pour a little olive oil on each slice of bread, then lay the slices of avocado and cucumber on top. Lightly season with salt. Add the slices of strawberry, drizzle with agave syrup and season with pepper. Scatter with the coriander leaves.

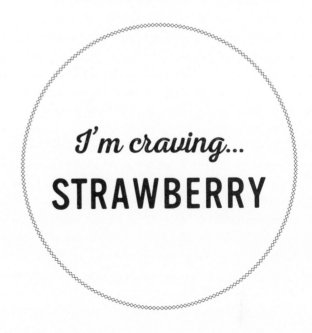

I'm craving...
STRAWBERRY

Strawberry soup
WITH MINT + BASIL

MAKES 2 BOWLS
PREPARATION TIME 10 MINUTES

250 g (9 oz) strawberries
5 sprigs mint
5 sprigs basil
60 g (2¼ oz) raw (demerara) or muscovado sugar
organic orange juice (optional)

Wash the strawberries and herbs. Dry them on paper towel. Cut the strawberries in two. Detach the mint and basil leaves. Set aside a few strawberries and a few leaves for garnish.

Blend the rest of the strawberries and herbs together in a food processor until smooth. Add the sugar, then process again on the highest setting for 30 seconds. Adjust the consistency if necessary with a little water or orange juice.

Pour the blended soup into pretty bowls. Set aside in the refrigerator and add some diced strawberry and a few basil and mint leaves at serving time.

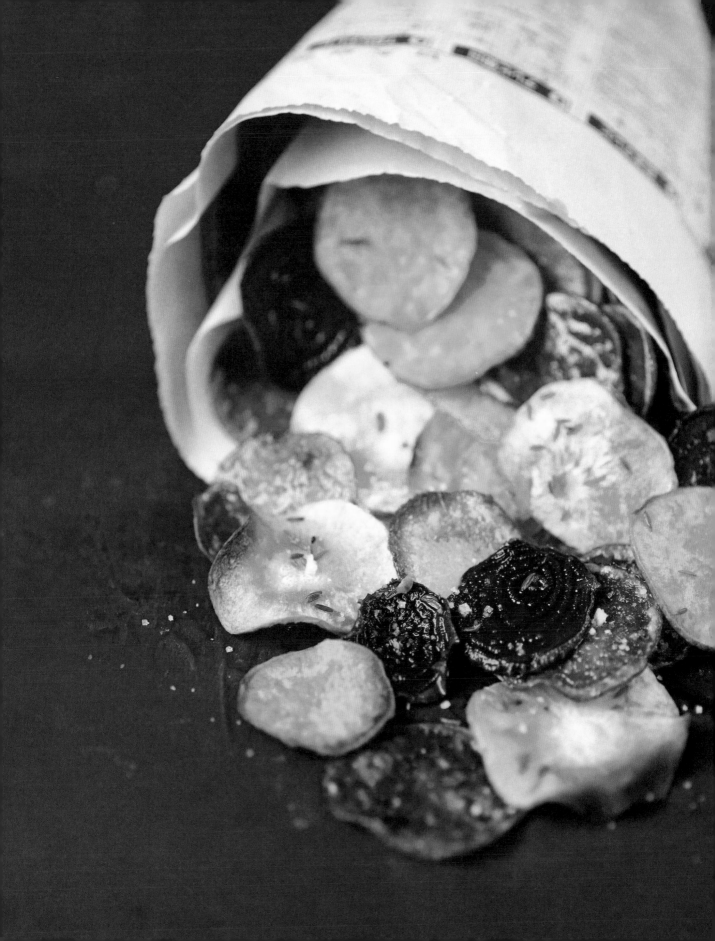

Sesame chips
WHITE + BLACK SESAME SEEDS

MAKES 1 LARGE BOWL OF CHIPS
PREPARATION TIME 20 MINUTES
COOKING TIME 10 MINUTES

1 free-range egg white
30 g (1 oz) plain (all-purpose) flour (or rice flour)
1 pinch of ground cumin
1 generous tablespoon olive oil
fine sea salt
2–3 tablespoons white and/or black sesame seeds

Preheat the oven to 180°C (350°F). Mix the egg white with the flour and cumin in a bowl. Whisk with a fork and add the olive oil in a thin stream.

Place small amounts of the batter on a baking tray lined with baking paper (or a silicone sheet), spreading them out a little with the back of a spoon: the batter should be very thin. Season with salt and add a pinch of white or black sesame seeds on each. Bake for about 10 minutes, or until the edges of the chips are golden. Let them cool, then remove the chips from the paper. Store in an airtight container.

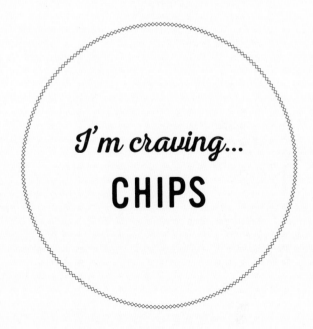

I'm craving...
CHIPS

Cheese crisps
WITH SPICES + PEAR

MAKES 1 LARGE BOWL OF CHIPS
PREPARATION TIME 15 MINUTES
COOKING TIME 10 MINUTES

250 g (9 oz) grated emmental or parmesan cheese
1 pinch of freshly ground pepper
1 pinch of cumin seeds
1 pinch of fennel or anise seeds
1 pinch of mild chilli powder or hot paprika
1 pear, peeled and diced

Preheat the oven to 180–200°C (350–400°F). Place small mounds, about 1 tablespoon, of grated cheese on a baking tray lined with baking paper. Sprinkle each with the spices. Bake in the oven for 10 minutes: the cheese should start to colour. Let the crisps cool before removing them from the paper. Serve with the diced pear.

TIP: To give these chips the curved shape of traditional crisps, lay them on a rolling pin while they are still warm and leave them to cool.

Oven chips
SWEET POTATO + PARSNIP + CARROT + PURPLE POTATO

MAKES 1 LARGE BOWL OF CHIPS
PREPARATION TIME 20 MINUTES
COOKING TIME 20–25 MINUTES

1 potato
1 sweet potato
1 parsnip
1 carrot
2 purple potatoes, such as congo, sapphire, purple gem
2 tablespoons olive oil
2 garlic cloves, peeled and crushed
paprika or mild chilli powder (optional)
salt flakes (e.g. Maldon) or fine sea salt

Preheat the oven to 210°C (425°F). Wash and dry all of the vegetables (keep the skin on if they are organic). Using a Y-shaped peeler or a mandoline, cut the vegetables into very thin slices. Place the vegetables in a zip-lock bag and add the olive oil, garlic and your choice of spice. Seal the bag and shake so that the vegetables are well coated with the seasonings.

Lay the vegetables slices flat on a baking tray lined with baking paper, without overlapping them. Bake for 20–25 minutes. Remove the chips from the oven, season with salt and let them cool. Store in an airtight container.

NOTE: Choose fresh, firm vegetables which will be easier to cut into very thin slices.

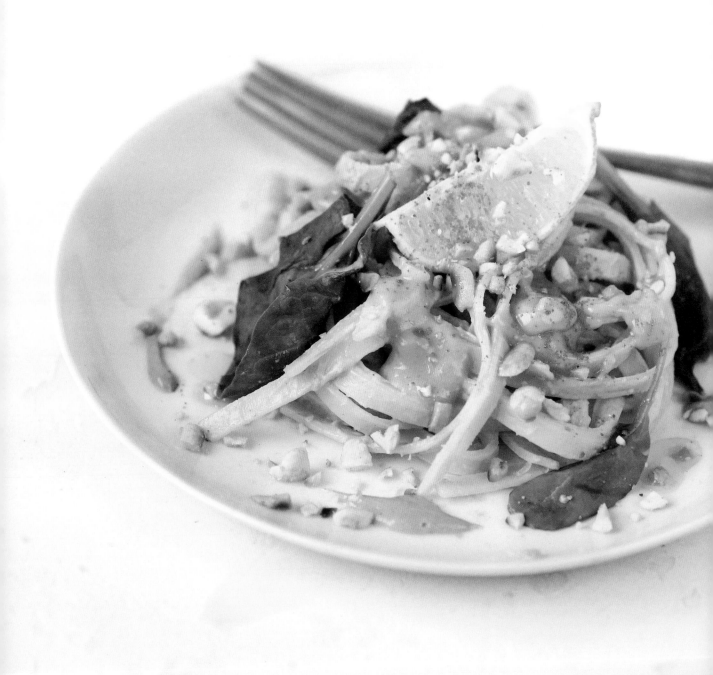

Satay noodles
WITH LIME + SPINACH

SERVES 2   PREPARATION TIME 10 MINUTES
COOKING TIME 10 MINUTES   RESTING TIME 5 MINUTES

200 g (7 oz) rice noodles
boiling water, as required
1 tablespoon shelled unsalted peanuts
2 handfuls baby spinach leaves
½ organic lime, plus wedges, to serve
1 pinch of hot paprika (optional)

Sauce

3 tablespoons home-made peanut butter (see below)
juice of ½ lime
1 garlic clove, peeled
1 tablespoon soy sauce (salt-reduced if possible)
2 tablespoons agave or maple syrup
1 pinch of chilli powder

Blend all the sauce ingredients together with 150 ml (5½ fl oz) water in a food processor until creamy. In a small saucepan, heat the sauce for 5 minutes over low heat.

Place the noodles in a large mixing bowl and cover with boiling water. Let them stand for 5 minutes, then drain.

Toast the peanuts for a few minutes in a dry frying pan, add the spinach and stir fry it very quickly. Mix the noodles with the sauce. Divide between shallow bowls and top with the spinach and toasted peanuts.

Serve with a wedge of lime and sprinkle with a little hot paprika if you like spicy dishes.

NOTE: You can also add a small, well-cooked chicken breast fillet.

Peanut butter
HOME-MADE

MAKES 1 JAR   PREPARATION TIME 2 MINUTES

250 g (9 oz) shelled peanuts. unsalted, unroasted
1 tablespoon grapeseed oil (or sesame oil)
1 pinch fine salt and/or 1 teaspoon agave syrup

Using a food processor, finely grind the peanuts on maximum power for 30 seconds. Add the oil, then process for another 30 seconds to form a paste. Add the salt and/or agave syrup and pulse a few more times. Place the peanut butter in a sterilised airtight glass jar. It will keep, refrigerated, for one week.

NOTE: You can also buy peanuts in their shells. To remove the skins easily, roast in a 180°C (350°) oven for 10 minutes, then rub between your fingers or in a clean tea towel (dish towel).

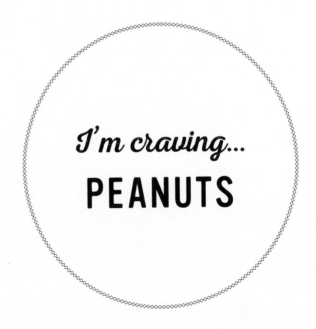

I'm craving...
PEANUTS

Mini peanut roughs

MAKES ABOUT 10 ROUGHS
PREPARATION TIME 10 MINUTES
COOKING TIME 15 MINUTES

250 g (9 oz/2½ cups) ground almonds and/or
   ground peanuts
250 g (9 oz/1⅔ cups) flour
125 g (4½ oz/1 cup) icing (confectioners') sugar
125 g (4½ oz) butter (or margarine), melted
1 free-range egg, beaten, plus 1 egg white
50 g (1¾ oz) shelled peanuts: unsalted and unroasted,
   roughly chopped

Preheat the oven to 180°C (350°). Combine the ground almonds, flour and icing sugar in a mixing bowl. Add the melted butter, then the beaten egg. Work together with your fingertips to make a smooth dough. In the hollow of your hand, using your fingertips shape the mixture into small balls, about 25 g (1 oz) each (the size of a walnut).

Set out a bowl with the egg white and a shallow bowl with the roughly chopped peanuts. Dip each ball in the egg white then roll it in the peanuts. Place the balls on a baking tray lined with baking paper and bake for about 15 minutes.

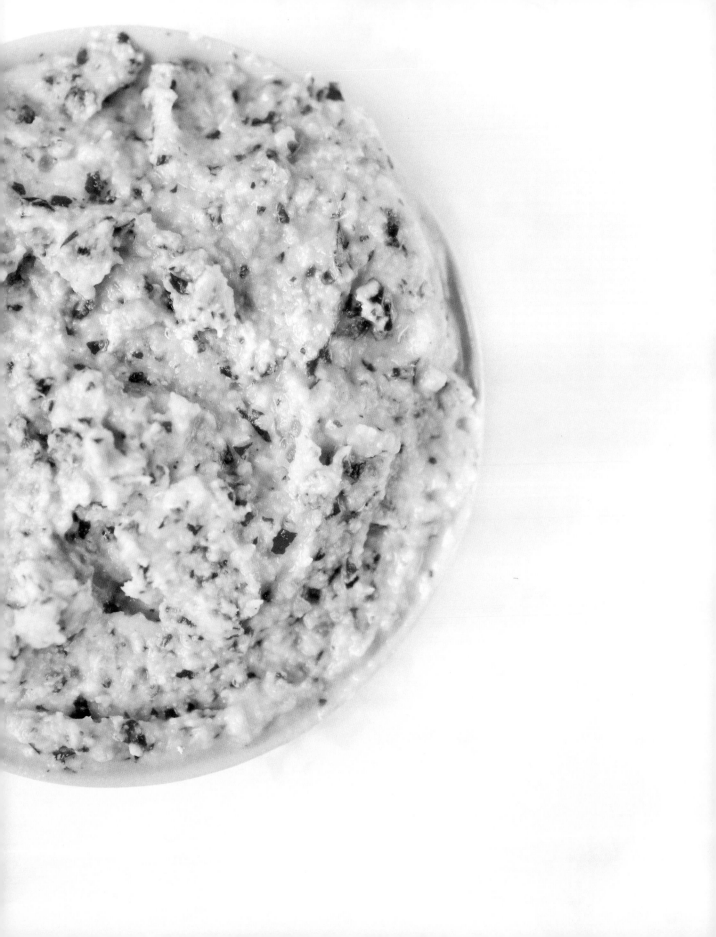

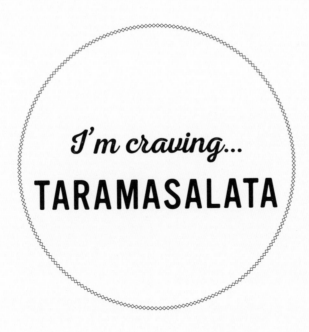

I'm craving...
TARAMASALATA

Crab taramasalata
with seaweed + semi-dried tomatoes + lemon

MAKES 1 BOWL
PREPARATION TIME 10 MINUTES
RESTING TIME 30 MINUTES

1 slice wholemeal (whole-wheat)
   bread, crust removed
2 tablespoons pasteurised milk
1 tin of shredded crab meat
   (145 g [5½ oz] drained weight)
1 semi-dried tomato in oil (or
   1 tablespoon ketchup)
juice of 1 organic lemon
2 teaspoons dried seaweed flakes
   (e.g. dulse flakes)
1 teaspoon salt

Place the slice of bread in a dish and cover with milk to soften. Using a food processor, pulse all of the ingredients for at least 30 seconds. Set aside in the refrigerator for 30 minutes before serving.

NOTE: Keeps for a maximum of 2 days in the refrigerator.

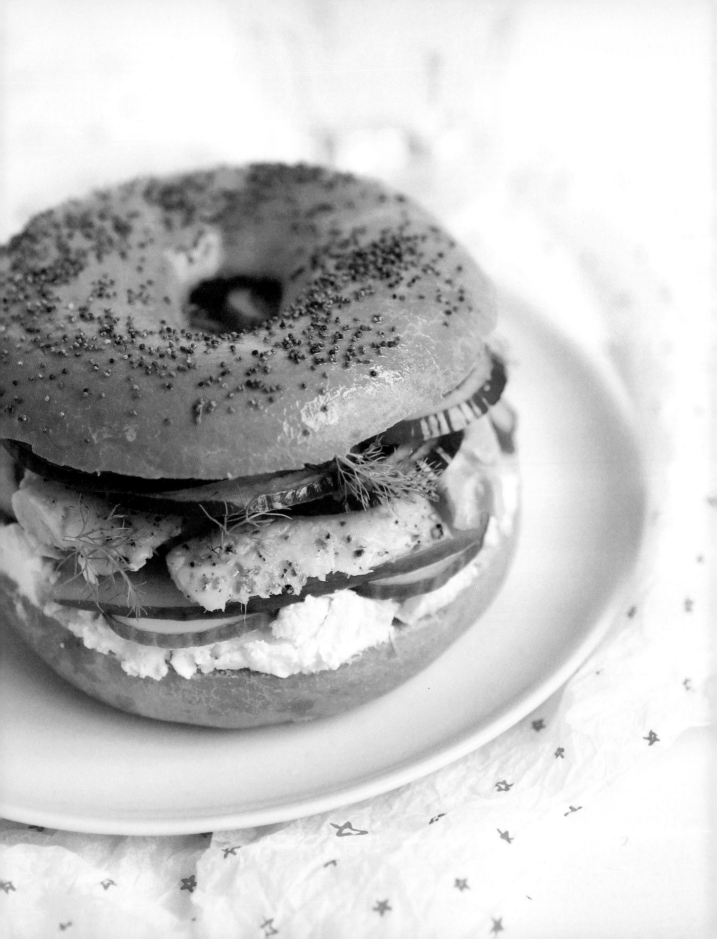

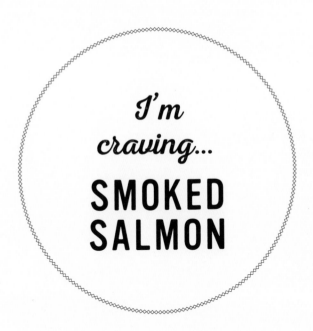

I'm craving...

SMOKED SALMON

Bagel
with tea-smoked salmon

SERVES 2
PREPARATION TIME 15 MINUTES
COOKING TIME 20–25 MINUTES

2 fillets of fresh salmon or 1 large
   300 g (10½ oz) fillet, not too
   thick, skin and bones removed
2 tablespoons olive oil
2 teabags of a smoky black tea,
   such as lapsang souchong
pinch of fine sea salt
2 bagels, cut in half

Filling
50 g (1¾ oz) cream cheese
½ cucumber, thinly sliced into rounds
sweet-sour pickles, thinly sliced
½ red onion, sliced into rings
2 sprigs dill, chopped

Wash the salmon fillets under cold water and dry them with paper towel. Brush both sides with olive oil. Place a sheet of foil in the bottom of a deep frying pan and place the tea on the foil. Pierce a sheet of baking paper with a fork and place it on top of the foil. Lay the salmon fillets on top and cook on a high heat for 20–25 minutes, covered: the salmon needs to be cooked right through. Season with salt and allow to cool.

Lightly toast the bagels. Spread them generously with cream cheese, top with the cucumber, pickles and salmon, cut into horizontal slices or strips. Add a few onion rings and some dill. Close the bagels and cut them in half before serving.

SMOKY FLAVOURS: Here are a few tips for creating smoky flavours: use smoked salt (from gourmet food stores), smoked butter (butter with smoked salt), smoky paprika.

COOKED SMOKED SALMON: You can eat smoked salmon if it is well cooked. Sear it in a hot, dry frying pan. Don't add salt to the recipe, because the smoked salmon will already be very salty.

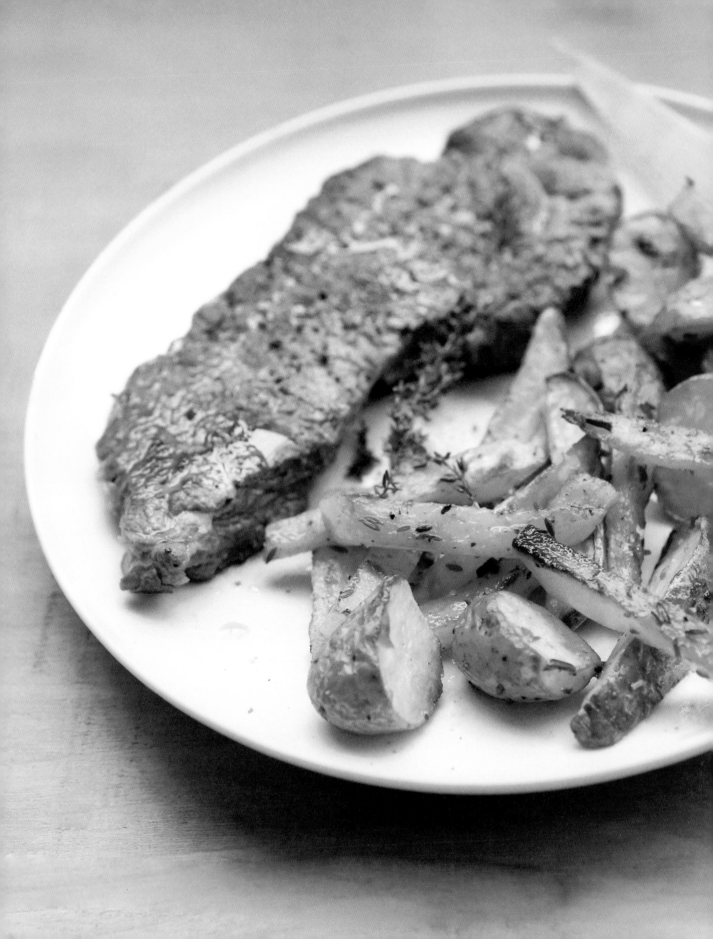

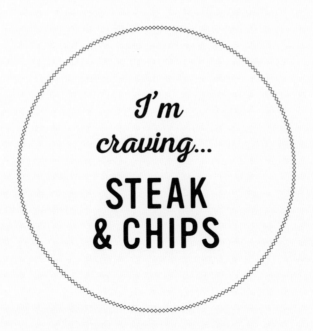

I'm craving...
STEAK & CHIPS

Light steak and chips
with paprika + fine sea salt

SERVES 4
PREPARATION TIME 25–30 MINUTES
COOKING TIME 30 MINUTES

Chips

5 or 6 large potatoes (such as bintje, charlotte or small fingerling potatoes)
2 tablespoons olive oil
1 teaspoon sweet paprika (optional)
2 teaspoons cumin seeds (optional)
2 sprigs rosemary, chopped (optional)
gomasio (sesame seed seasoning)

Steak

2 slices of beef fillet, sirloin or rump steak
1 tablespoon olive oil (optional)
2 pinches of fine sea salt, freshly ground pepper

Preheat the oven to 200°C (400° F). Cut the potatoes into chips or wedges. Peel the potatoes beforehand if cutting into chips (but not for wedges). Dry them well with paper towel. Soak the chips in salted water for 10 minutes. Drain and dry again to remove as much starch as possible. Place the chips in a zip-lock bag. Add the olive oil, spices and/or rosemary, if using, and shake the bag well to coat the potatoes.

Spread out the chips on a baking tray lined with baking paper. Bake for about 25 minutes, stirring half way through the cooking. Season with gomasio when they come out of the oven.

Heat a cast-iron grill pan or a non-stick frying pan over high heat. Once it is very hot (but not smoking), lay the steaks in the pan without adding any fat. Turn the meat over after 3 minutes: it should be seared — this happens very quickly. Cook for a further 3 minutes, or until cooked to medium. If necessary, you can also lightly oil the grill pan by brushing with a tablespoon of olive oil. Season and serve with the chips.

COMMENT: Choose a lean, good quality cut of steak, which will stay tender even when cooked to medium.

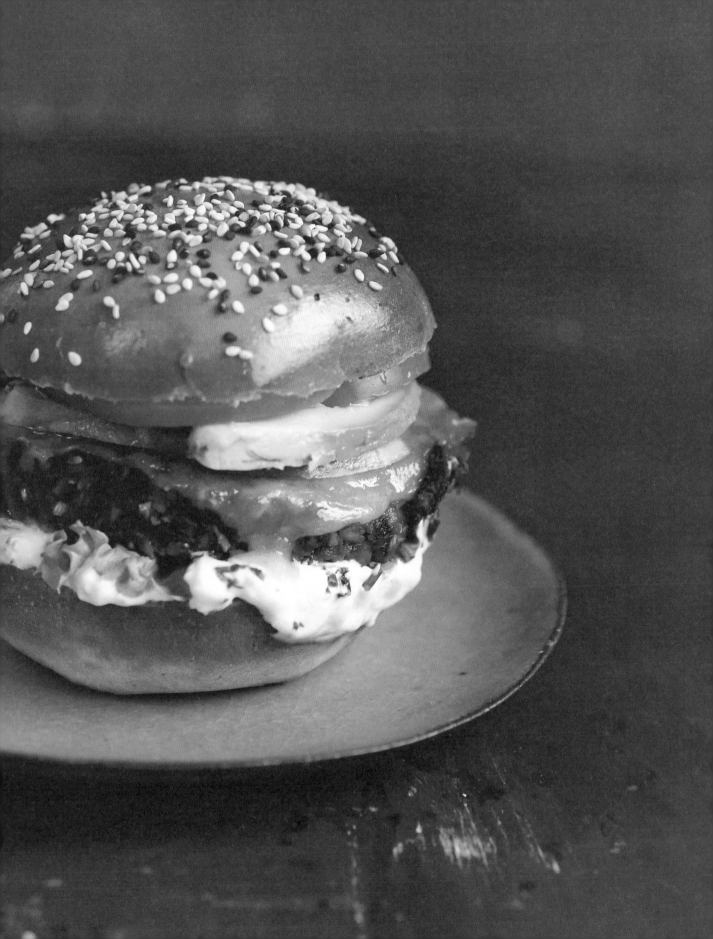

Veggie burger
BEETROOT + AVOCADO + CHEDDAR

MAKES 4 HAMBURGERS
PREPARATION TIME 25 MINUTES
COOKING TIME 25 MINUTES – RESTING TIME 20 MINUTES

2 carrots, grated
1 raw beetroot (beet), grated
1 small onion, chopped, plus extra whole rings, to serve
100 g (3½ oz/1 cup) rolled oats
2 free-range eggs
½ bunch of chives, finely chopped
1 teaspoon salt, freshly ground pepper
2–3 drops Tabasco sauce
4 slices cheddar cheese
4 leaves lettuce
1 avocado, thinly sliced
1 tomato, sliced into rounds
4 home-made buns (see page 162) or store-bought
    hamburger buns

Yoghurt sauce
125 g (4½ oz/1 small tub) Greek yoghurt + 1 teaspoon
honey-mustard sauce + 2 spring onions (scallions),
sliced + ½ bunch snipped chives + salt, pepper

Preheat the oven to 200°C (400°F). Mix the carrots
with the beetroot, onion, oats, eggs and chives.
Season and add a few drops of Tabasco. Mix with
a fork until smooth. Let the mixture rest, refrigerated,
for 20 minutes. Shape into four balls and flatten slightly.
Place on a baking tray lined with baking paper. Bake
for 15–18 minutes. Five minutes before the end of
cooking time, place a slice of cheddar on each patty.

Mix the sauce ingredients together. Season.

Warm the buns in the oven for 5 minutes, then spread
with a little sauce. Add the lettuce, the veggie burger
with melted cheese, avocado slices, onion rings and
a slice of tomato.

Chicken burger
WITH PARMESAN + YOGHURT SAUCE

Cut 4 thick chicken fillets in half horizontally. Cover
with plastic wrap and flatten with a rolling pin. Dip
in a mixture of beaten egg, paprika, chilli, Tabasco, salt
and pepper, then in breadcrumbs flavoured with thyme.
Brown them on each side in a frying pan in olive oil.
Assemble the burger with the yoghurt sauce, lettuce
and shavings of parmesan cheese.

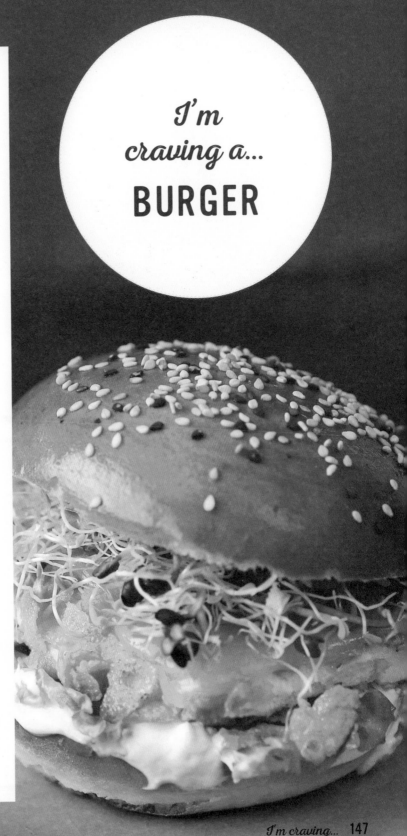

*I'm
craving a...*
BURGER

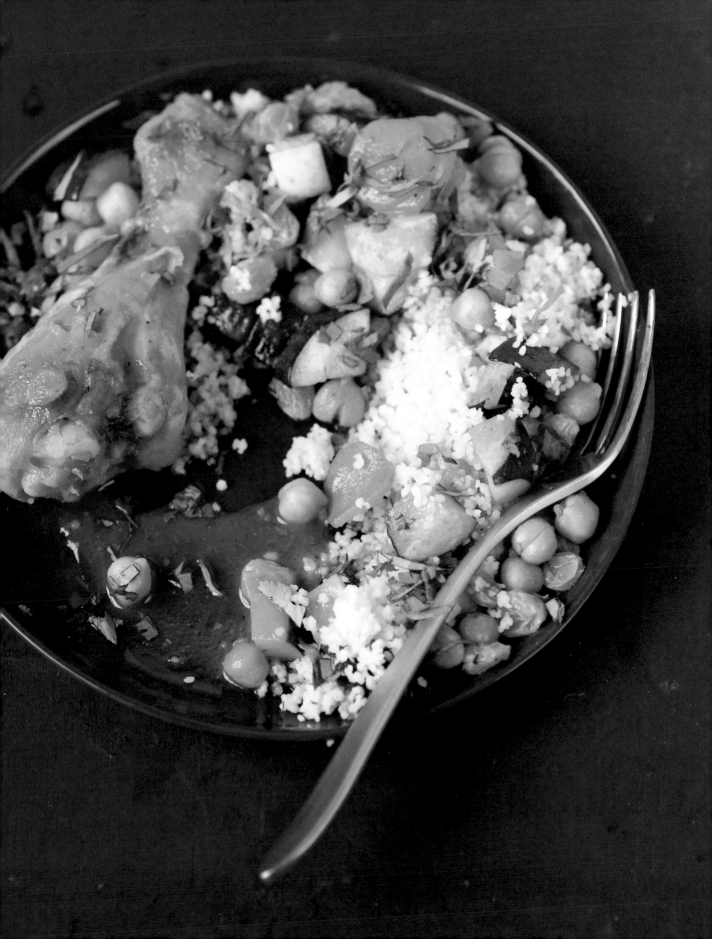

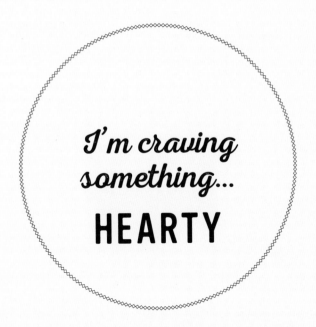

I'm craving
something...
HEARTY

Express tagine
chicken + carrot + zucchini + chickpeas

SERVES 2
PREPARATION TIME 15 MINUTES
COOKING TIME 30 MINUTES–1 HOUR

2 tablespoons olive oil
2 or 4 chicken drumsticks,
　skin removed
½ teaspoon salt, pepper
dried thyme (or oregano)
1 pinch of mild chilli powder
1 carrot, peeled and sliced into rounds
1 zucchini (courgette), cubed
60 g (1¼ oz) chickpeas, cooked
　and drained
2 tablespoons tomato paste
　(concentrated pureé)
ras-el-hanout spice mix (or a mixture
　of cumin, ginger and turmeric)
30 g (1 oz) raisins
500 ml (17 fl oz/ 2 cups) water
160 g (5¾ oz/¾ cup) wholemeal
　(whole-wheat) couscous (or quinoa
　or burghul [bulgur])
chopped parsley and coriander
　(cilantro), to serve

Heat the olive oil in a deep frying pan over high heat and add the drumsticks. Season with salt and pepper and brown on all sides. Add a little thyme and mild chilli powder; mix together. Add the carrot, zucchini, chickpeas, tomato paste, spices, raisins and water. Simmer for about 45 minutes, covered, until the vegetables are cooked.

Near the end of the cooking time, place the couscous in a large bowl. Add 2 ladles of broth from the pan, cover with plastic wrap and leave for 5 minutes, or until the liquid is absorbed. Season with salt.

To serve, divide the couscous between two bowls. Add the drumsticks, vegetables and broth and sprinkle with the chopped herbs.

TIP: Try adding a small, lean grilled merguez or spicy chorizo sausage.

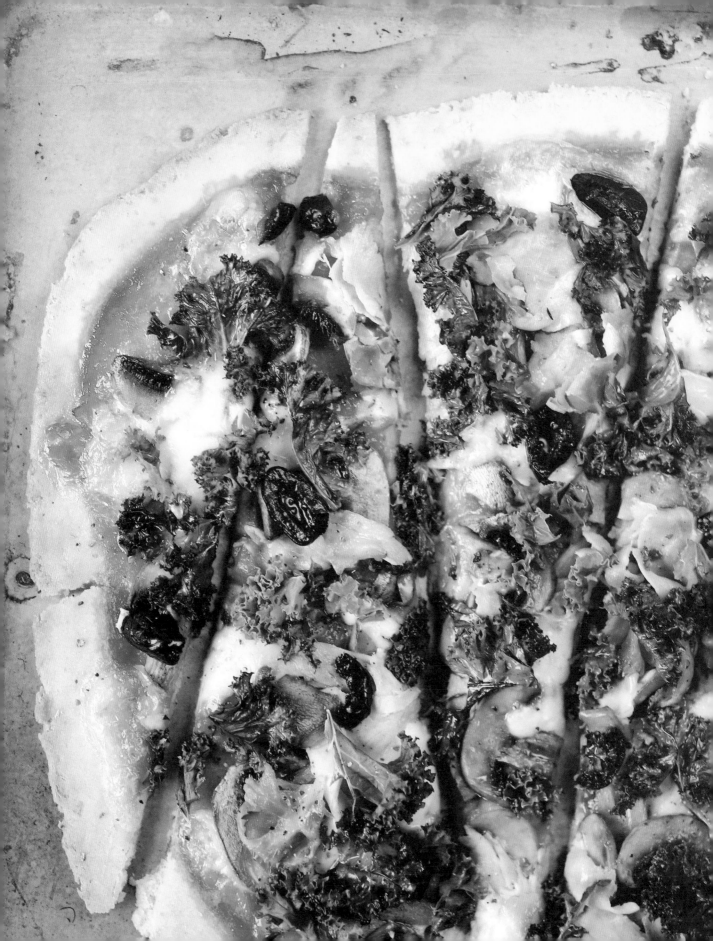

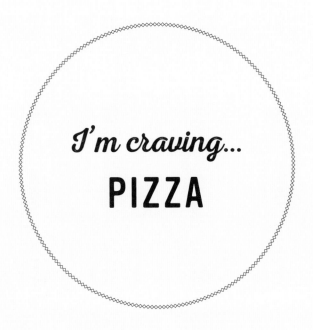

I'm craving...
PIZZA

Pizza mamma
mushrooms + mozzarella + kale

MAKES 1 PIZZA
PREPARATION TIME 15 MINUTES
COOKING TIME 10–12 MINUTES
RESTING TIME 30 MINUTES–2 HOURS

1 wholemeal (whole-wheat) pizza
 base (see page 163)
200 ml (7 fl oz) tomato passata
 (or tomato pasta sauce)
2 pinches of dried oregano
200 g (7 oz) fresh mushrooms,
 thinly sliced
2 thin slices ham, shredded
1 ball mozzarella cheese, sliced
 into rounds
5–6 black olives
1 small handful kale, shredded
1 handful well-washed rocket
 (arugula) (optional)
1 bunch basil or flat-leaf (Italian)
 parsley (optional)

Preheat the oven to 250°C (500°F). Roll the pizza dough out thinly on a floured surface.

Spread the tomato passata over the base, sprinkle with dried oregano, then evenly distribute the mushrooms, shredded ham, mozzarella, olives and kale. Bake for 10–12 minutes.

Take the pizza out of the oven. Scatter over a good handful of rocket and fresh herbs, if using, and serve.

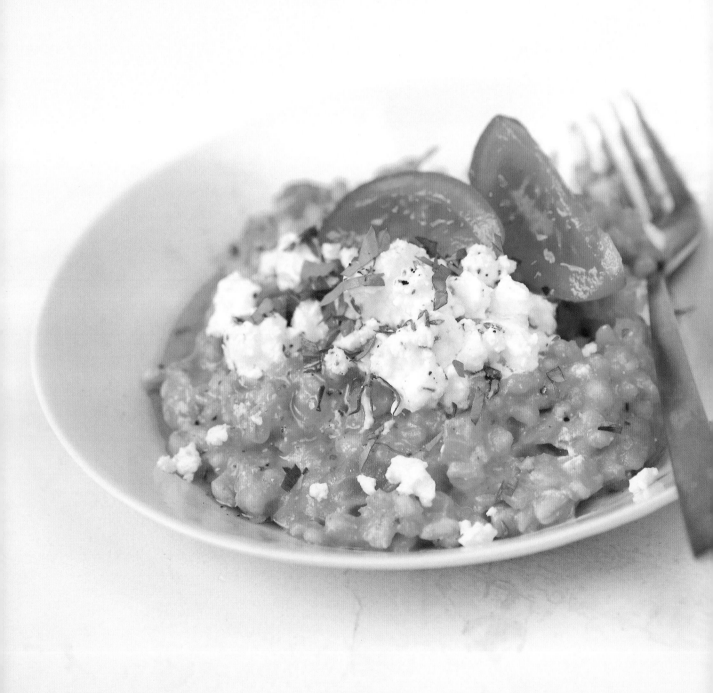

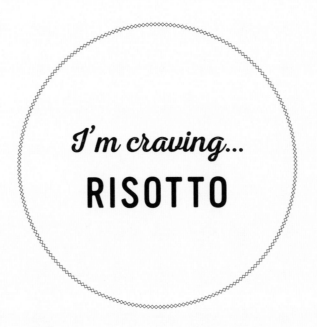

I'm craving...
RISOTTO

Barley risotto with tomato

SERVES 4
PREPARATION TIME 15 MINUTES
COOKING TIME 50 MINUTES

200 g (7 oz) pearl barley (or
   short-grain rice)
2 tablespoons olive oil, for frying,
   plus 100 ml (3½ fl oz) extra
2 small French shallots, finely sliced
4 garlic cloves, sliced
2 small celery stalks, cut into 5 mm
   (¼ inch) slices
½ teaspoon paprika
1 bay leaf
4 sprigs thyme (or rosemary)
4 strips organic lemon rind
700 ml (24 fl oz) vegetable stock
300 ml (10½ fl oz) tomato passata
400 g (14 oz) tinned peeled tomatoes
salt and freshly ground pepper
30 g (1 oz) unsalted butter
300 g (10½ oz) pasteurised feta
   cheese (or fresh goat's cheese,
   or ricotta)
1 teaspoon cumin (seeds or ground)
fresh oregano (or basil) leaves,
   to garnish

Rinse the barley under running cold water and drain.

In a deep frying pan, heat the 2 tablespoons of olive oil over medium heat and gently sauté the shallots. Add the garlic and celery. Soften them for 5 minutes, stirring. Add the paprika, bay leaf, thyme and lemon rind and mix together. Add the barley and cook for 1 minute, then add the vegetable stock, passata and peeled tomatoes. Season and stir well to combine. Bring to the boil, then lower the heat and simmer for 45 minutes, covered, over a low heat: the barley is cooked when it is tender and the liquid is almost completely absorbed. Add the butter and mix well.

In a small bowl, use a fork to mix the feta with the cumin and extra olive oil. Serve the barley risotto topped with the crumbled feta, garnished with fresh oregano leaves.

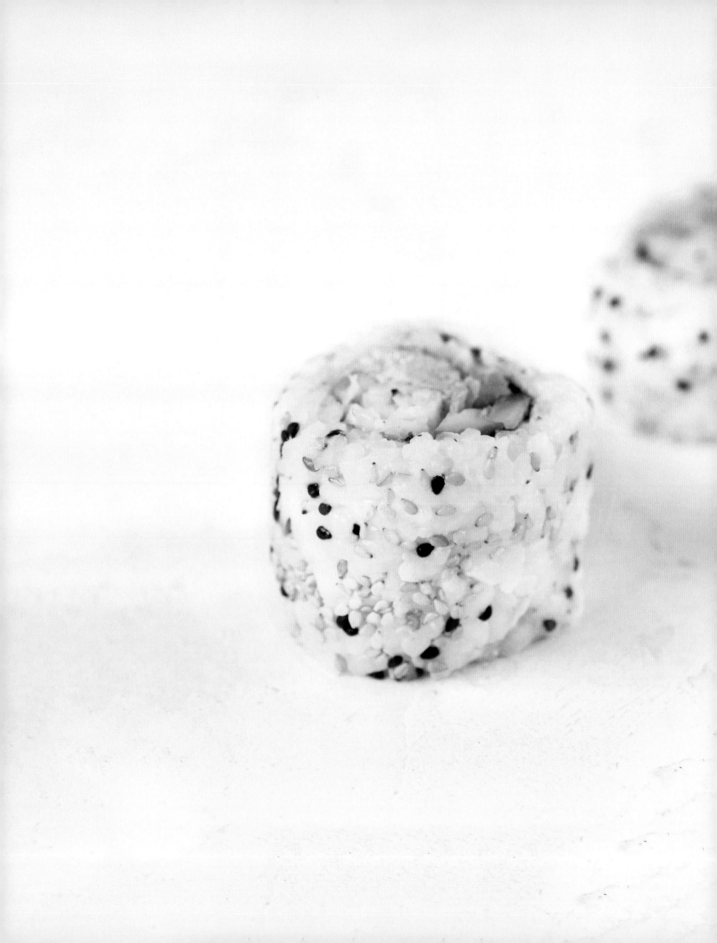

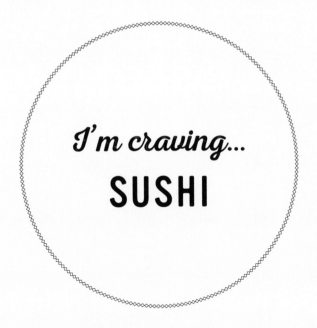

I'm craving...
SUSHI

California rolls
cooked tuna + cucumber + avocado

MAKES 12 ROLLS
PREPARATION TIME 30 MINUTES
COOKING TIME 10 MINUTES
RESTING TIME 30 MINUTES

Rice
200 g (7 oz/1 cup) sushi rice
30 ml (1 fl oz) rice vinegar
15 g (½ oz) sugar
1 pinch of fine salt

Filling
160 g (5¾ oz) tinned tuna or salmon,
    drained
2 tablespoons mayonnaise
2 sheets nori seaweed
2 pinches of sesame seeds
1 teaspoon cumin (seeds or ground)
½ carrot, peeled and grated
¼ radish, grated
¼ cucumber, cut into sticks
½ avocado, thinly sliced

Accompaniments
salt-reduced soy sauce
wasabi paste
pickled ginger

Cook the rice as per the instructions on the packet. In a bowl, mix the tuna with a tablespoon of mayonnaise.

Set out a small bowl of lukewarm water. Cover a bamboo mat with plastic wrap and lay a sheet of nori on top. Moisten your fingers so the rice doesn't stick to them and spread the rice over the nori sheet in a fairly thin layer. Sprinkle with sesame seeds. Turn over the sheet of nori so that the rice is underneath and the nori is on top. Lay some carrot, radish, tuna, cucumber and avocado across the middle of the sheet. Roll up tightly from the bottom, using the plastic wrap to make an even roll. Make the other roll and rest them for 30 minutes in the refrigerator.

Slice each roll into 6 pieces with a large knife. To stop the knife from sticking, dip it into warm water between each cut. Serve the sushi rolls with salt-reduced soy sauce, wasabi and pickled ginger.

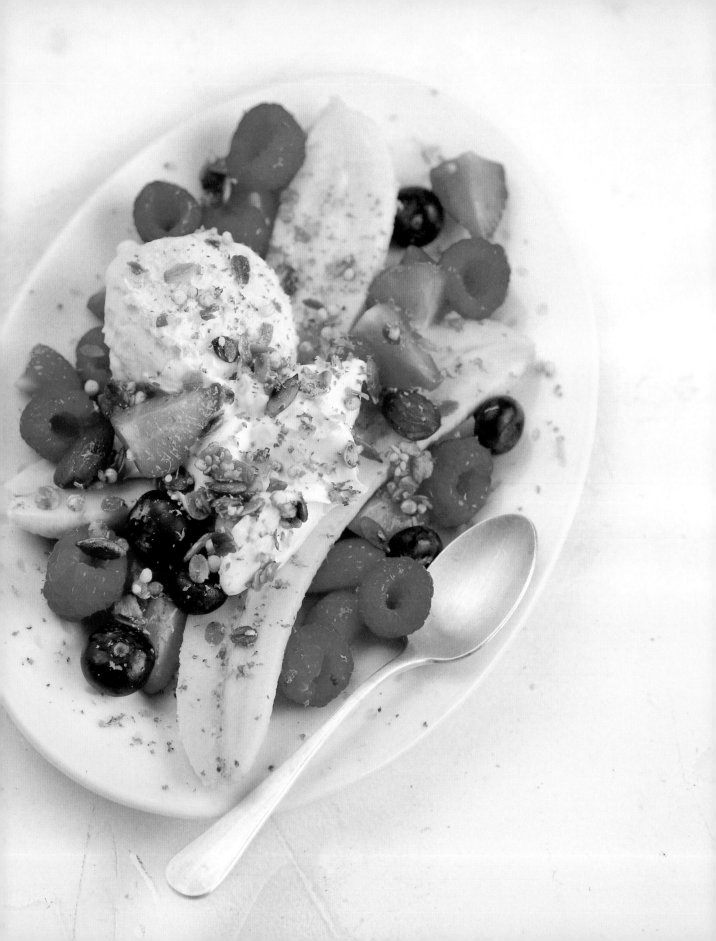

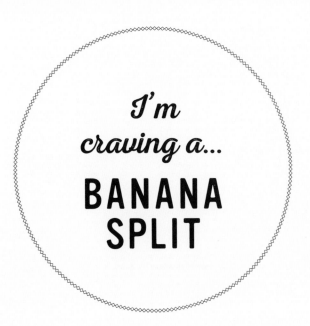

I'm craving a...
BANANA SPLIT

Fruity banana split
with coconut whipped cream

SERVES 2
PREPARATION TIME 10 MINUTES
RESTING TIME 15 MINUTES

200 ml (7 fl oz) tinned coconut milk
   (or, better, coconut cream, from
   health food stores)
1 tablespoon icing (confectioners')
   sugar
zest of ½ untreated organic lime
2 bananas
1 handful blueberries
1 handful strawberries and raspberries
4 scoops frozen yoghurt (see
   page 159) (or vanilla ice cream)
4 tablespoons home-made granola
   (see page 30) (or a few chopped
   walnuts)
3 squares chocolate

For the whipped cream, open the tinned coconut milk and lift off the thick, solid, creamy part on top. Chill this coconut cream in a glass mixing bowl with the beater attachments of an electric beater in the freezer for 15 minutes.

Remove from the freezer, add the icing sugar and beat until the coconut cream mixture has doubled in volume. Gently mix the lime zest into the whipped coconut cream.

Halve the bananas and add the remaining fruit, whole or in pieces. Arrange 2 scoops of ice cream in a dish, then sprinkle with the granola. Add a quenelle, or scoop, of whipped coconut cream and grate the chocolate on top.

HOT/COLD VARIATIONS: Cook the half bananas for a few minutes in a frying pan with a tablespoon of coconut oil. Make a chocolate sauce (see page 127) and pour over the dessert.

TIP: If you want to make a quenelle of whipped cream or pipe it, place the cream in the freezer for 2 hours before use.

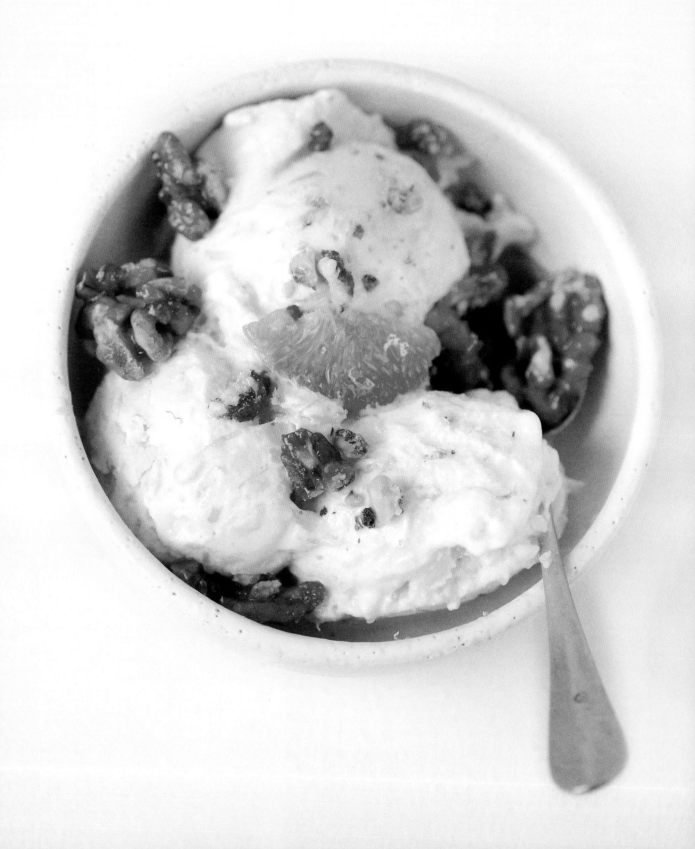

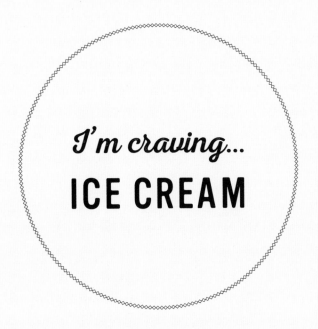

I'm craving...
ICE CREAM

Frozen yoghurt
ginger + grapefruit + crunchy walnuts

MAKES 2 OR 3 BOWLS
PREPARATION TIME 15 MINUTES
RESTING TIME 3 HOURS 30 MINUTES

1 organic pink grapefruit
300 g (10½ oz) plain Greek-style
    yoghurt
4–5 tablespoons agave syrup or
    icing (confectioners') sugar
2 cm (¾ inch) fresh ginger, peeled
    and grated

Topping
100 g (3½ oz) shelled walnuts
100 ml (3½ fl oz) maple syrup

Peel the grapefruit, removing the white pith as well, and take out the segments. Mix together the yoghurt with the agave syrup in a bowl and add the grapefruit and ginger. Mix together with a fork.

Pour the mixture into an ice-cream maker, churn it for 20–30 minutes and place it in the freezer. If you don't have an ice-cream maker, pour the mixture into a loaf tin and place it in the freezer for 3 hours, mixing every 45 minutes with a fork.

Meanwhile, heat the walnuts in a frying pan for 1 minute over medium heat. Pour the maple syrup over and let it caramelise, stirring to coat the walnuts well. Cool the nuts on a sheet of baking paper.

Add 2 scoops of frozen yoghurt to each bowl and sprinkle with caramelised walnuts.

EXPRESS VERSION: The day before, place the fruit of your choice in the freezer. On the day, blend the fruit directly with the yoghurt and add the topping.

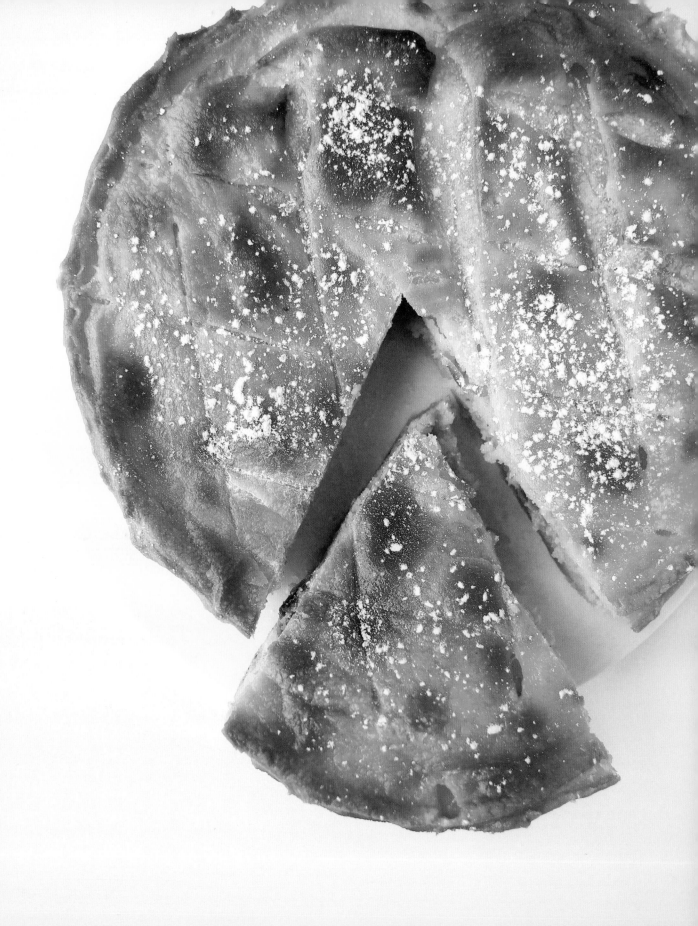

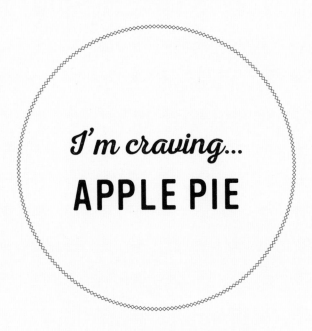

I'm craving...
APPLE PIE

Galette des reines
with petit-suisse + apple

MAKES 1 GALETTE
PREPARATION TIME 20 MINUTES
COOKING TIME 25–30 MINUTES
RESTING TIME 1 HOUR 15 MINUTES

1 quantity petit-suisse puff pastry
   (see page 163)

Filling
50 g (1¾ oz) butter, softened
100 g (3½ oz/½ cup) raw
   (demerara) sugar
1 free-range egg
100 g (3½ oz/1 cup) ground almonds
1 drop bitter almond essence
150 g (5½ oz) apple/pear purée
3 dried dates, finely chopped
2 drops liquid vanilla extract
1 teaspoon cinnamon

Glaze
1 egg, beaten
2 tablespoons pasteurised milk
1 teaspoon raw (demerara) sugar

Mix the butter with the sugar in a bowl using a whisk or a fork. Add the egg and mix well until smooth. Add the ground almonds, bitter almond extract, apple/pear purée, dates, vanilla and cinnamon. Rest the filling, covered, in the refrigerator for 30 minutes so it firms up.

Preheat the oven to 200°C (400°F).

Divide the pastry into two equal portions. Set one aside in the refrigerator, wrapped in plastic wrap. Roll out the other portion on a floured work surface. Use it to line a round pie or tart dish, no more than 26 cm (10½ inches) in diameter. Place it in the refrigerator.

Roll out the second pastry portion into a round about 2 cm (¾ inch) larger than the dish.

Spread the filling over the pastry base, making sure to leave a 1 cm (½ inch) border. Brush the edge of the pastry with beaten egg. Lay the second round of pastry on top, and carefully seal the edges of the 2 rounds together with your fingers. Glaze the galette by brushing over the rest of the beaten egg mixed with the milk and raw sugar. Score the top of the galette with a diamond or ear-of-wheat pattern.

Bake the galette for 25–30 minutes.

Basics
FOR THE MUM-TO-BE
Here are the pregnancy alternatives to basics used for day-to-day cooking: healthy, light, quick.

LEMON VINAIGRETTE
An ultra-quick and very easy vinaigrette recipe with lemon to fight nausea and nutrient-packed tahini.

Blend the juice of ½ lemon with 2½ tablespoons of water, 1 tablespoon tahini or white miso, 1 teaspoon cider vinegar, 1 pinch each of salt and pepper in a jar. You can also add 1 tablespoon olive or canola oil for a slightly richer version. Keeps for 3 days in the refrigerator.

FROMAGE BLANC SAUCE
A delicious and very digestible sauce because it doesn't contain any oil. Perfect with raw vegetables.

Mix 4 tablespoons of fromage blanc (or quark or labneh) with the juice of ½ lemon, 1 teaspoon honey-mustard sauce, and 5 finely chopped chives. Season and mix together well with a fork.

SUPER-SPICY KETCHUP
Without any colours or preservatives, home-made ketchup is very healthy: just tomato and spices. An ideal condiment for pregnant women.

Place in a saucepan: 750 ml (26 fl oz/3 cups) tomato passata (or purée), 2 tablespoons of cider vinegar, 1 tablespoon of Worcestershire sauce, 1 tablespoon of honey, 3 tablespoons cornflour (cornstarch), 1 teaspoon sweet (or smoky) paprika, 1 teaspoon salt, 1 teaspoon cinnamon, 1 tablespoon light brown sugar. Heat over a low heat for 20 minutes, stirring with a whisk: the sauce should thicken. Adjust the seasoning if necessary and pour into a clean glass bottle. Keeps for 1 week in refrigerator.

EXPRESS BÉCHAMEL
This béchamel sauce is very easy to make. It is less rich and heavy than ready-made béchamel sauces.

Gradually whisk 500 ml (17 fl oz/2 cups) pasteurised milk into 50 g (1¾ oz/⅓ cup) plain (all-purpose) flour in a small mixing bowl. Add a drop of olive oil. Pour into a saucepan and heat gently. Stir continuously with a whisk until it reaches the desired consistency. Season generously and add some nutmeg.

MARINADE FOR MEAT
Ideal for marinating chicken, pork or lamb.

Place in a zip-lock bag: ½ crushed garlic clove, the juice and zest of 1 organic lemon, 125 g (4½ oz/1 small tub) plain yoghurt, 2 tablespoons olive oil, 1 teaspoon of honey-mustard sauce, 1 teaspoon ras-el-hanout spice mix, 1 teaspoon of salt and a little pepper or chilli. Add the meat, seal the bag and shake well. Marinate for 1 hour in the refrigerator. Remove the meat, reserving the marinade, and cook it in the oven, in a frying pan or on a hotplate. Towards the end of the cooking time, you can pour the marinade over the meat to coat it or make a sauce, ensuring it simmers for at least 5 minutes before serving. For salmon, add a handful of chopped herbs, e.g. coriander (cilantro), dill.

BLINIS (MAKES 10)
Buckwheat blinis for more nutrients and low-GI carbohydrates.

Whisk 2 eggs with a pinch of salt. Add 500 ml (17 fl oz/2 cups) milk, beating continuously. Gradually add 100 g (3½ oz/¾ cup) buckwheat flour and 100 g (3½ oz/⅔ cup) wholemeal (whole-wheat) flour with 2 teaspoons of baking powder. Let the mixture rest for 30 minutes in the refrigerator. Add a knob of butter to a non-stick frying pan, make small rounds of batter in the pan and let them cook for 3 minutes. When small bubbles form on the surface of the blinis, turn them over to cook for another 1–2 minutes.

BUNS (MAKES 4 OR 5)
Much better than store-bought ones.

In a mixing bowl, mix together 360 g (12¾ oz) plain (all-purpose) flour with 200 ml (7 fl oz) lukewarm milk. Add 14 g (½ oz/ 4 teaspoons) of dried yeast or 20 g (¾ oz) fresh yeast, then 3 teaspoons of sugar, ⅓ teaspoon of salt, 2 teaspoons lemon juice and 1 knob of butter. Knead everything for 5 minutes, in a mixer or by hand: the dough should come away easily from the sides of the bowl or your fingers.

Divide the dough into four or five balls, about 160 g (5¾ oz) each. Place them on a baking tray lined with baking paper. Let them rest at room temperature for 50 minutes. Fifteen minutes before the end of the proving time, preheat the oven to 210°C (410°F). Slash the top of each ball a few times, dab a little water on top with your finger, then sprinkle with sesame, poppy or sunflower seeds. Place a small bowl of water on the bottom of the oven to create steam and give the buns a good crust. Bake the buns for about 15 minutes: they should be nice and golden.

PICKLES (MAKES ONE 1 LITRE JAR)
For the first-trimester cravings for sour things.

Heat 125 ml (4 fl oz/½ cup) sherry vinegar or rice vinegar with 3 tablespoons of salt, 75 g (2¾ oz/⅓ cup) of sugar and 250 ml (9 oz/1 cup) water in a saucepan, stirring, for 5 minutes. Turn off the heat once the sugar and salt have completely dissolved. Cut 3 small cucumbers, 1 small fennel bulb, 5 pink radishes and ¼ cauliflower into small pieces (florets, rounds, cubes). Place them in a sterilised 1 litre (35 fl oz/4 cups) jar and pour over the pickling liquid. Cool the pickles before closing the jar and place them in the refrigerator for 24–48 hours before opening. The pickles keep for 3–4 weeks in the refrigerator.

WHOLEMEAL PIZZA DOUGH
Thanks to the wholemeal spelt flour, this dough contains more low-G.I carbohydrates than ready-made pizza bases.

Blend 1 teaspoon powdered yeast with 1 teaspoon of lukewarm water and leave it to froth for 5 minutes. Knead together 125 g (4½ oz) plain (all-purpose) flour, 125 g (4½ oz) wholemeal (whole-wheat) spelt or rice flour, 125 ml (4½ fl oz/½ cup) lukewarm water, 2 tablespoons olive oil, 1 tablespoon milk, ½ teaspoon salt, and the yeast. Rest the dough 30 minutes to 2 hours, covered, near a source of heat, before rolling it out thinly.

EXPRESS SHORTCRUST PASTRY
Very quick to make, this home-made pastry recipe, with no butter or egg, works for all quiches and savoury tarts.

Pour 250 g (9 oz/1⅔ cups) wholemeal (whole-wheat) flour, a pinch of salt, 100 ml (3½ fl oz) olive oil, and about 2½ tablespoons of lukewarm water into a mixing bowl and work together with your fingertips. The dough should be very pliable; adjust the amount of flour or water, if necessary. Shape into a smooth ball. Cover with plastic wrap and set aside in the refrigerator until using or roll it out straight away.

RUSTIC SWEET SHORTCRUST PASTRY
This sweet pastry is very easy to make. It is delicious as a case for fruit tartlets.

Mix together 200 g (7 oz/1⅓ cups) wholemeal (whole-wheat) flour, 60 g (2¼ oz) raw (demerara) sugar and 1 pinch of salt in a bowl. Add 60 g (2¼ oz) butter and rub in with your fingertips until the dough looks like a crumble mixture. Mix in 1 egg yolk and 2 tablespoons cold water: the dough should form a smooth ball. Roll the pastry dough out on a floured surface and set it aside for 15 minutes in the refrigerator before using.

WHOLEMEAL SWEET PIE CRUST
Thanks to the wholemeal and chestnut flours, this pastry contains more complex carbohydrates. The almond butter also gives it lots of nutrients. It is suitable for all sweet tarts.

Mix together 150 g (5¼ oz/1 cup) wholemeal (whole-wheat) flour, 120 g (4¼ oz) chestnut flour, 1 pinch of salt, 1 tablespoon raw sugar and ½ teaspoon bicarbonate of soda (baking soda) in a mixing bowl. Melt 100 g (3½ oz) butter with 80 g (2¾ oz) almond butter and 3 tablespoons of milk. Gradually mix the wet mixture into the dry mixture, then add 1 egg yolk. Work the dough until it forms a very smooth ball. Cover with plastic wrap and set it aside for 1 hour in the refrigerator before using.

PUFF PASTRY WITH PETITS-SUISSE
A quick, light and calcium-rich puff pastry, made using petit-suisse cheese.

Combine 140 g (5 oz) plain (all-purpose) flour and 120 g (4¼ oz) petits-suisses (or thick Greek yoghurt), then mix in 2½ tablespoons of water: the dough should be smooth but not sticky; add a little flour if necessary. Cover with plastic wrap and let the dough rest for 30 minutes in the refrigerator. Roll out the dough with a rolling pin on a floured surface. Dot the dough with 50 g (1¾ oz) butter, cut into small cubes, and fold it over on itself like a wallet. Work it a little with your fingertips to spread out the butter, then return it to the refrigerator for 15 minutes. Take it out, roll it out again and fold it over again like a wallet. Let it rest for another 15 minutes.

OAT BRAN CRUMBLE MIXTURE
Crumbles with bran have the advantage of having less fat. They make delicious express crumbles with fresh or cooked fruit.

Using your fingertips, mix together 50 g (1¾ oz) softened butter (unsalted or semi-salted), in pieces, with 50 g (1¾ oz/¼ cup) light brown sugar, 70 g (2½ oz) oat bran and 1 pinch of cinnamon in a mixing bowl: the dough should be like breadcrumbs and form clumps. Add a little more bran or water if necessary. Sprinkle this mixture over fruit and bake in the oven for 20 minutes at 180°C (350°F).

Recipe index

Craving a flavour

Sometimes you become obsessed with a specific flavour... sweet, spicy, fresh... Here's how to dip into this book as the craving takes you.

Craving an ingredient

Acknowledgements

I would like to thank all the pregnant women around me (and there are lots of them!), who confided their own CRAVINGS to me! Béatrice, Katya, Susanne, Sophie, Marianne, Aurélie, Sabina. All of them convinced me that this book was a good idea, I can't wait to see your little cuties …

Thank you to the whole maternity team at Maternité des Lilas, Pascale Delage especially, who supported me during my pregnancy. What an adventure! Thank you to the whole Marabout team, Pauline, Rose-Marie, Emmanuel, Elisabeth, for their support and the trust they put in me on every one of my projects. Thanks in advance to Anne and Émilie who will work to make sure all the mums-to-be will know about this book! I also thank Aurélie for her support during the writing process. It wasn't easy, right in the middle of maternity leave!

Thank you to the photo team who pitched in to make this book pretty while I was bottle feeding. Thanks Émilie and Eléa for your work, you were the best.

To my mum friends who gave me good advice all throughout my pregnancy.

To my family who is always there when I need them, thank you.

To my sweetheart, the father of my daughter, who I will never be able to tell enough how much I love him.

And my daughter, Lou, my finest work!

Published in 2017 by Murdoch Books, an imprint of Allen & Unwin
First published by Marabout in 2015

Murdoch Books Australia
83 Alexander Street
Crows Nest NSW 2065
Phone: +61 (0) 2 8425 0100
Fax: +61 (0) 2 9906 2218
murdochbooks.com.au
info@murdochbooks.com.au

Murdoch Books UK
Ormond House
26–27 Boswell Street
London WC1N 3JZ
Phone: +44 (0) 20 8785 5995
murdochbooks.co.uk
info@murdochbooks.co.uk

For Corporate Orders & Custom Publishing, contact our Business Development Team at salesenquiries@murdochbooks.com.au.

Publisher: Corinne Roberts
Designer: Olivia Design
Cover design: Vivien Valk
Photographer: Émile Guelpa
Translator: Melissa McMahon
Editor: Karen Lateo
Production Manager: Rachel Walsh

Text and design copyright © Hachette Livre (Marabout) 2015
The moral rights of the author have been asserted.

A cataloguing-in-publication entry is available from the catalogue of the National Library of Australia at nla.gov.au.

ISBN 978 1 74336 812 1 Australia
ISBN 978 1 74336 815 2 UK

A catalogue record for this book is available from the British Library.

Printed by C & C Offset Printing Co. Ltd., China

IMPORTANT: The content presented in this book is meant for inspiration and informational purposes only. The purchaser of this book understands that the author is not a medical professional, and while best efforts have been made to ensure the accuracy of the information, the information contained within this book is not intended to replace medical advice. Pregnant and breastfeeding women should follow the advice of their obstetrician, GP or midwife. The author and publisher claim no responsibility to any person or entity for any liability, loss, or damage caused or alleged to be caused directly or indirectly as a result of the use, application, or interpretation of the material in this book.

OVEN GUIDE: You may find cooking times vary depending on the oven you are using. For fan-forced ovens, as a general rule, set the oven temperature to 20°C (70°F) lower than indicated in the recipe.

MEASURES GUIDE: We have used 15 ml (3 teaspoon) tablespoon measures.